Disability, Spaces and Places of Policy Exclusion

Geographies of disability have become a key research priority for many disability scholars and geographers. This edited collection, incorporating the work of leading international disability researchers, seeks to expand the current geographical frame operating within the realm of disability. Providing a critical and comprehensive examination of disability and spatial processes of exclusion and inclusion for disabled people, the book uniquely brings together insights from disability studies, spatial geographies and social policy with the purpose of exploring how spatial factors shape, limit or enhance policy towards, and the experiences of, disabled people.

Divided into two parts, the first part explores the key concepts to have emerged within the field of disability geographies, and their relationship to new policy regimes. New and emerging concepts within the field are critically explored for their significance in conceptually framing disability. The second part provides an in-depth examination of disabled people's experience of changing landscapes within the onset of emerging disability policy regimes. It deals with how the various actors and stakeholders, such as governments, social care agencies, families and disabled people traverse, these landscapes under the new conditions laid out by changing policy regimes. Crucially, the chapters examine the lived meaning of changing spatial relations for disabled people.

Grounded in recent empirical research, and with a global focus, each of the chapters reveals how social policy domains are challenged or undermined by the spatial realities faced by disabled people, and expands existing understandings of disability. In turn, the book supports readers to grasp future policy directions and processes that enable disabled people's choices, rights and participation. This important work will be invaluable reading for students and researchers involved in disability, geography and social policy.

Karen Soldatic is International Researcher in Disability Policy Studies at the University of New South Wales, Australia and Adjunct Research Fellow of the Centre of Human Rights Education, Curtin University, Australia.

Hannah Morgan is Lecturer in Disability Studies in the Department of Sociology and member of the Centre for Disability Research at Lancaster University, UK.

Alan Roulstone is Professor of Disability Studies, University of Leeds, UK and has held senior posts in a number of universities.

T0270699

Routledge Advances in Disability Studies

Disability, Spaces and Places of Policy Exclusion

Edited by
**Karen Soldatic, Hannah Morgan and
Alan Roulstone**

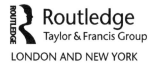

LONDON AND NEW YORK

First published 2014 by Routledge

2 Park Square, Milton Park, Abingdon, Oxfordshire OX14 4RN

52 Vanderbilt Avenue, New York, NY 10017

Routledge is an imprint of the Taylor & Francis Group, an informa business

First issued in paperback 2019

Copyright © 2014 selection and editorial material, Karen Soldatic, Hannah Morgan and Alan Roulstone; individual chapters, the contributors

The right of the editor to be identified as the author of the editorial material, and of the authors for their individual chapters, has been asserted in accordance with sections 77 and 78 of the Copyright, Designs and Patents Act 1988.

All rights reserved. No part of this book may be reprinted or reproduced or utilised in any form or by any electronic, mechanical, or other means, now known or hereafter invented, including photocopying and recording, or in any information storage or retrieval system, without permission in writing from the publishers.

Notice:
Product or corporate names may be trademarks or registered trademarks, and are used only for identification and explanation without intent to infringe.

British Library Cataloguing in Publication Data
A catalogue record for this book is available from the British Library

Library of Congress Cataloguing in Publication data
  Disability, spaces and places of policy exclusion / edited by Karen Soldatic,
  Hannah Morgan, Alan Roulstone.
    pages   cm. – (Routledge advances in disability studies)
  ISBN 978-0-415-85480-1 (hardback) – ISBN 978-0-203-73984-6 (ebook)
  1. People with disabilities – Government policy.   2. Public spaces.   I. Soldatic, Karen.
  II. Morgan, Hannah.   III. Roulstone, Alan, 1962–
  HV1568.D56947 2014
  362.4'04561–dc23
  2013050694

ISBN: 978-0-415-85480-1 (hbk)
ISBN: 978-0-367-34577-8 (pbk)

Typeset in Times
by Out of House Publishing

Contents

vi   *Contents*

Contributors

Claire Edwards is Lecturer in the School of Applied Social Studies, University College Cork, Ireland. Her background is in urban and cultural geography and social policy. Her research interests include the participation of disabled people in society and the disability rights agenda; urban regeneration and the effectiveness of urban policy, particularly in terms of its ability to provide benefit for excluded communities; and the politics of knowledge production, and the relationship between social research and policy. Her most recent research has been concerned with exploring how patients' organisations (and specifically, organisations representing families of children with ADHD) seek to influence the production of medical knowledge about health conditions, and the barriers disabled people face in accessing the criminal justice system as victims of crime in Ireland. Theoretically, Claire is interested in exploring cross-disciplinary linkages between geography, social policy and sociology, and in particular, examining the potential of social and geographical theory to illuminate understandings of disability and health and illness in society. Claire previously worked as a Senior Research Officer at the Department for Work and Pensions and Disability Rights Commission in the UK.

Kayleigh Garthwaite is a post-doctoral research associate in the Department of Geography, Durham University. She has been involved in a range of research projects around poverty, social exclusion, chronic illness, disability, health inequalities and worklessness. Kayleigh has published in the field of disability studies, social policy, youth studies and public health. Currently, Kayleigh is working on a five-year project involving an urban ethnography of health inequalities in the borough of Stockton on Tees, UK, drawing on sociological and anthropological theory to examine how health inequalities are embodied in lived experiences.

Shaun Grech is a sociologist currently based at Manchester Metropolitan University, UK and editor-in-chief of the international journal, *Disability and the Global South* (DGS). His critical and interdisciplinary research addresses disability and poverty as a project of decolonising pedagogy and praxis. He has published in leading academic journals, is author of the book *Disability, Poverty and the Global South: Critical Reflections from Guatemala* (Palgrave

Macmillan), and recently co-edited the book *Inclusive Communities: A Critical Reader* (Sense Publishers). Shaun is also an activist working in collaboration with local DPOs to provide emergency health care to disabled people in extreme poverty in Guatemala, an action research project run on behalf of Integra, a Maltese non-profit organisation.

Chris Grover is a senior lecturer in social policy at Lancaster University, UK. His research interests primarily focus upon social security policy. He has written extensively on the political economy of social security policy through focussing upon policies to subsidise low paid employment and the application of conditionality to social security benefits. In this context he has examined various aspects of the recent development of income replacement social security benefits for disabled people in the UK. His most recent work focuses upon the economic and moral imperatives of the use of loans within poor relief and social assistance policy.

Edward Hall is Lecturer in Human Geography at the University of Dundee. He has undertaken a series of research projects on the social geographies of disability, with a particular focus on learning disability. The projects have examined the positions and experiences of disabled people in employment; the social exclusion and inclusion of people with learning disabilities; the 'personalisation' of social care for disabled people; and the potential of the creative arts to develop belonging for people with learning disabilities. These projects have been funded by the ESRC, Nuffield Foundation, Scottish Government and the Royal Geographical Society. Edward has published widely in leading journals including *Environment and Planning A*, *Geoforum* and *Disability and Society*, and co-edited with Vera Chouinard and Rob Wilton *Towards Enabling Geographies: Disabled Bodies and Minds in Society and Space* (Ashgate, 2010). In 2012–13 he co-ordinated an ESRC Seminar Series, 'Rethinking Learning Disability', bringing together academics from a range of disciplines, people with learning disabilities, social care practitioners, and policy makers.

Andrea Hollomotz came to academia from a social work and care background. She is interested in examining how social policy and practice affect the everyday lives of disabled people. Her PhD focused on the social creation and construction of sexual 'vulnerability' of adults with learning difficulties. This explored more general themes around sex and sexuality, self-advocacy and choice making. More recently, Hollomotz has become increasingly interested in criminal justice issues and forensic practices with people with learning difficulties. She is currently involved in an EU funded collaborative project on disabled children's access to justice. For a list of the most significant publications, see: www.sociology.leeds.ac.uk/about/staff/hollomotz.php.

Rob Imrie is Professor of Sociology in the Department of Sociology at Goldsmith College London. He is presently directing a European Research Council Advanced Investigators Grant project (2013 to 2016) about universalism and universal design, and is co-ordinating a series of Economic and Social

Research Council funded seminars about designing inclusive environments. His most recent book, co-authored with Emma Street, is *Architectural Design and Regulation* (Wiley & Blackwell, 2011).

Hannah Morgan is Lecturer in Disability Studies in the Department of Sociology and member of the Centre for Disability Research at Lancaster University. She is the lead organiser of the biennial international disability studies conference held at Lancaster since 2003. The conference attracts over 220 delegates from a wide variety of countries. Hannah is also a member of the editorial board of the international journal *Disability and Society* and since May 2012 is also the book reviews editor. Hannah's research interests focus on the spatial dimensions of disability in relation to varying service models of support. She has published widely and recently co-edited, in collaboration with Prof Alan Roulstone, a special edition of *Social Work Education* (2012).

Andrew Power is Lecturer in Human Geography in the Department of Geography and Environment at the University of Southampton. Prior to coming to Southampton he worked as a post-doctoral researcher at the Centre for Disability Law and Policy at the National University of Ireland Galway. Andrew's research interests focus on the spatial dimensions of disability, independent living, personalisation and welfare reform. He has published widely in the geographies of disability and disability studies including recent papers in *Social Science and Medicine* (2013) and *Disability and Society* (2013) as well as two recent books, *Landscapes of Care: Comparative Perspectives on Family Caregiving* (2010) with Ashgate and *Active Citizenship and Disability: Implementing the Personalisation of Support* (2013) with Cambridge University Press.

Donna Reeve is a disability studies theorist who has been researching and writing about psycho-emotional disablism for ten years. Her general interests also include identity, the body and social theory with a focus on the lived experience of disability. She is an Honorary Teaching Fellow at Lancaster University.

Alan Roulstone is Professor of Disability Studies, University of Leeds and has held senior posts in a number of universities. He is a sociologist who has for the last 25 years been producing sociologically-underpinned contributions to disability studies and social policy research, writing and teaching. He has been involved in a wide range of international research projects around adult health and social care, ageing, disability, disablist hate crime, social exclusion, transitions to work and adulthood, chronic illness, new technologies and social futures, older people, and disability law. Funders include SCIE, the Leverhulme Trust, Joseph Rowntree Foundation, Department of Health, Disability Rights Commission (now EHRC), European Commission, Economic and Social Research Council, Regional Development Agencies, and UNESCO. He aims to link the academy, activist organisations and policy influencers. He has produced over 60 isbn/issn publications in the fields of disability, equality, crime, work, law, human rights and employment policy.

Karen Soldatic is an international researcher in disability policy studies at the University of New South Wales, Sydney and was recently recognised for her research on changing international disability policy frameworks with a British Academy International Visiting Fellowship (2011–12). Her research work has been published in leading international journals including: *International Journal of Population Research* (2012), *Scandinavian Journal of Disability Studies* (2013), *Social Work Education* (2012) and *Societies* (2012). Karen is also an adjunct research fellow of the Centre of Human Rights Education, Curtin University.

Jon Warren is a sociologist who is currently Senior Research Associate in Public Health Policy, based at the Wolfson Research Institute, Department of Geography, Durham University. His research interests are centred on work, employment, the work-life interface and the industrial history of the north east of England. Jon conducts methodologically innovative research and is currently involved with projects using Qualitative Comparative Analysis (QCA) and Visual methods. He has published work in the fields of disability studies, public health policy and the sociology of work. Jon was previously part of the School of Applied Social Sciences at Durham where he taught Sociology and Social Work. Jon undertook his doctoral studies on work–life relations in the call centre industry in the UK and India. Prior to coming to Durham Jon was a lecturer in Community and Youth Studies at Sunderland University and also a researcher for the Office for National Statistics.

Acknowledgements

The set of papers included in this volume emerged from a two-day workshop held at Lancaster University in 2012. Thanks to the extensive support provided by the Centre for Disability Research (CeDR), Lancaster University, disability researchers engaging with the geographies from across the UK, Ireland and Australia were able to attend and present preliminary findings from their research. Engaging and lively debate ensued and this volume represents the re-working of these papers as a result of collegial and rigorous discussions on the relationship between disability, space and place, and policy, particularly given the rise and intensification of 'austerity' politics locally and internationally.

The two-day forum was also the outcome of a British Academy International Visiting Fellowship awarded to Karen Soldatic and Carol Thomas. The team would like to thank Carol for encouraging and supporting Karen's application and for her ongoing support for the project. Additional thanks go to the Centre for Human Rights Education, Curtin University, who supported Karen's trip to Lancaster and also the follow-up support with manuscript finalisation. On this note, special thanks to Rebecca Eckert, who has come to this project with the responsibility to 'order the disorder' that an international edited volume brings.

Acronyms

ACOSS	Australian Council of Social Services
BC	British Columbia
BOCG	Brothers of Charity Galway
BSI	British Standards Institution
CBR	Community Based Rehabilitation
CMP	Condition Management Programme
COSLA	Convention of Scottish Local Authorities
CRDP	Convention on the Rights of Persons with Disabilities
DDA	Disability Discrimination Act
DLA	Disability Living Allowance
DoH	Department of Health
DR	Dial-a-Ride
DRC	Disability Rights Commission
DSP	Disability Support Pension
DWP	Department for Work and Pensions
EHRC	Equality Human Rights Commission
ESA	Employment Support Allowance
ESRC	Economic and Social Research Council
FAO	Food and Agricultural Organization
FG	Focus Group
GP	General Practitioner
HCPs	Health Care Professionals
HMSO	Her Majesty's Stationery Office
IB	Incapacity Benefit
IBSEN	Individual Budgets Evaluation Network
IFAD	International Fund for Agricultural Development
INT	Interview
JSA	Job Seekers Allowance
LAC	Local Area Co-ordinator
LTH	Lifetime Homes
MDG	Millennium Development Goal
ODI	Office for Disability Issues
ODPM	Office of the Deputy Prime Minister

OECD	Organisation for Economic Co-operation and Development
PCP	Person-centred Planning
PIP	Personal Independence Payment
PWD	People with Disabilities
SCLD	Scottish Consortium for Learning Disability
SDS	Self-Directed Support
TfA	Transport for All
TfL	Transport for London
UN	United Nations
UNESCO	United Nations Educational, Scientific and Cultural Organization
WCA	Work Capability Assessment
WHO	World Health Organisation

Introduction: disability, space, place and policy

New concepts, new ideas, new realities

*Alan Roulstone, Karen Soldatic and
Hannah Morgan*

Introduction

Geographies of disability and spatial geographies have rightly taken their place
in the wider canon of disability research and disability studies. That disablement
is a spatial issue seems at one level a truism; however a key driver for this edited
collection is the perception that the wider panoply of geographical insights
on disability, embodiment and the emplaced body has not been applied that
systematically to the forms of policy and legal exclusions experienced by disabled
people in contemporary society. Indeed notions of policy and space rarely sit
together save for a small number of descriptive readings of building regulations
and anti-discrimination legislation and guidance. Policy has not to date been
conceptualised as a spatial phenomenon. Policy is often reified as natural and fixed,
at least once it is formulated. We argue that policy spaces and their relationship
to physical, psycho-social and ontological spaces afforded to disabled people
need to be central to our understanding of social space and enabling/disabled
society. Social policy both emanates from and continually remakes the spaces or
constraints that directly influence disabled people's life opportunities. To reflect
such new insights we aim to respond to such an absence of critical attention and
to engage more fully notions of disability, policy and space. Both policy and law
embody constructions of 'right' bodies and minds and thus frame current and
future social possibilities for disabled people. Space, for example, being able to
occupy freely certain public, private or even 'taboo' spaces, is heavily inscribed
with disablist notions of just what is possible given disabled people's capability,
capacity and reason.

In the chapters that follow we draw on the commissioned writings of geographers, sociologists, policy and disability studies academics to provide a range
of insights into the nature, reproduction and challenge to the spatial and policy-
inscribed exclusion of disabled people. We take as our cue a number of important
preceding works that have been published in what might be framed as disability
geographies, and which help set the scene for the work that follows. Such works
focus on matters as diverse as physicality and commodification (Gleeson, 1999;
Hansen, 2002), disability and spatial justice (Butler and Parr, 1999; Kitchin, 1998),
the spatial dynamism and boundaries of disabled bodies (Haraway, 1991), ableism

(Imrie, 1996; Kumari-Campbell, 2009), and the fluid biographical identity that negotiates, traverses and navigates a range of complex social spaces, places and landscapes (Chouinard *et al.*, 2010; Crooks *et al.*, 2008; Imrie, 2007; Maddern and Stewart, 2010). The chapters that follow aim to expand the current geographical frame of reference operating within the realm of disability; intersecting three critical, yet often contrasting, ideas, of disability, space and place, *and* social policy regimes. Through critical conceptual analysis and based on empirical insights, the chapters explore how current policy and legal regimes re/map, re/frame and re/shape divergent spatial relations and realities for disabled people. In this context, the spatial is not confined to the material and structural alone. A key feature of a number of chapters that follow are their attempts to disclose the diverse ways disability and spatial relations are constructed symbolically, culturally and materially. Thus, the book challenges readers to consider the 'multifaceted spatial dimension' of social policy for disabled people and the imposition of altering policy regimes that confine, override or disguise the spatial dimension of social life for disabled people. For example, changing welfare regimes not only have profound consequences in terms of their financial settlements for disabled people, but represent a profound-reframing of belonging, legitimacy and selfhood.

The chapters included within this volume therefore provide a critical and comprehensive examination of disability and spatial processes and their impact on the contemporary exclusion or inclusion of disabled people. While this reflects the growing increase in academic attention on issues of disability and critical policy and practice (Oliver and Barnes, 2012; Roulstone and Prideaux, 2012), the book extends current theoretical and empirical discussions and debates in the area via pivoting this analysis around 'the spatial' and 'the geographical' and their links to and from policy systems. As the chapters together suggest, there is now a compelling need to critically review, conceptualise and explore the ways in which policy and spatial constructions re/shape and re/frame disabled people's experience of the social world in a number of country contexts internationally. To distil the uneven and differentiated effects of the inter-relationship of these dynamics upon disabled people, a number of empirical spheres are explored, such as the law, policy and programmes from countries as diverse as Australia, Canada, Guatemala, UK and Ireland. The chapters explore public and private space as typically conceptualised within the realm of disability geographies as differing spheres of social life, while engaging with policy and law that shape sexual, personal, economic and legal choices across a range of varying scales. Each of the chapters reveals how these social policy domains are challenged or undermined by the spatial realities faced by disabled people.

Space then is not simply the end product of, or a material challenge to, policy; policy-making itself attempts to construct spaces and places via opportunities that may previously have been closed off to disabled people individually or as a social category. A good example of such processes are the Disability Discrimination Acts developed in the United States, UK and Australia – these statutes were in part bound up with both the potential redefinition of spatial options (adjustments to environments for example) and the reshaping of policy space (such as the involving of disabled people within the disability policy process). Yet, in turn, these progressive initiatives can be undermined by pre-existing, enduring or new/emerging spatial barriers to environments (structural, cultural and material) and the policy process. Rather than see policy as a process or quantum of social imperatives, the spatial dimension facilitates the connection of innovative disability studies ideas that explore policy as spatial redefinition and as a space of contested social priorities.

The chapters contained within Part II of the book draw upon recent empirical research that has sought to explore the interstice of disability, policy change and spatial relations. These rich empirical chapters provide a window into disabled people's experiences of changing relations of space and place with the onset of policy changes that govern these spatial settings. The chapters distil the ways in which disabled people negotiate and traverse these varying environments, and the resultant impacts and effects upon disabled people's lives materially, discursively and symbolically. The insights emerging from Part II of the book highlight to the readership that while disability policies may appear to have as their target the category of people known as disabled people, in fact, these policies have a broader lived reality in the way they transform the spatial dimension of disability.

The compilation of the work presented within this volume aims to locate discussions about disability, disablism/disablement and disabled people within the wider spatial turn occurring within the social sciences, acknowledging the disability lacuna within existing spatial discussions and debates, and the limited emphasis on space and place in mainstream disability studies.

The book structure and chapters explained

The book is made up of two parts. First, Part I, a conceptual section, aims to provide a state-of-the-art picture of the ways in which disability is constructed and reconstructed in policy assumptions. This part will provide the reader with critical and searching appraisals of space and disability in a way that better underpins a reading of Part II of the book. Part II aims to draw on recent empirical evidence from a range of country contexts on how policy is premised on certain constructions of disability and how policy serves to constrain or support disabled people in their daily lives. It explores how space is experienced in given policy contexts. This introductory chapter provides a general overview and orientation to the book and rehearses a range of theoretical, conceptual and empirical issues to arise in the wider chapters. Chapter 1 by Imrie explores the multiple intersections between disability, public policy and geography. Its overarching observation is that there is limited explication about the interrelationships between the lives of disabled people and the geographies of public policy, or the intrinsically spatialised nature of state policy regimes. The chapter explores how fruitful lines of inquiry, between geography, social policy and disability studies, may be the basis for enhancing understanding of the impact of policy regimes on disabled people. The chapter begins by recognising the significance of changes in the nature of contemporary citizenship, underpinned by the re/evaluation of what productive bodies are or ought to be. Developing Ong's (2006) observation, that people's citizenship is based upon their marketable skills, the chapter suggests that the human worthiness of disabled people is, increasingly, being discredited in a context whereby welfare policy reform is placing the onus on self-active and self-starting individuals as the basis of a 'good' society. The techniques and technologies of governing, that seek to re/shape the nature of citizenship, are part of the formation of policy regimes that are unstable and malleable. These characteristics of policy regimes are shaped by their inherently geographical nature, in which, as Imrie argues, the fortunes of disabled people have to be understood as indissoluble from the interstices between space, place and policy.

In Chapter 2, Edwards provides a searing critique of the way in which sexual offences legislation delimits personal and spatial freedoms for people with learning difficulties in Ireland. She draws on debates emanating from the sub-discipline of 'legal geography' to explore how law shapes understandings of disabled people as victims of (sexual) crime by regulating disabled bodies and their interaction with public/private space. It draws on contestation over a particular piece of criminal law in Ireland, Section 5 of the Criminal Law (Sexual Offences) Act 1993, which in seeking to protect people with learning disabilities from sexual abuse also places restrictions on people with learning disabilities to engage in consenting sexual relationships. Through examining this legislation, the chapter unpicks the 'law-space nexus' (Blomley, 1989) by illustrating how law engages in boundary work to imagine victim and offender identities in different spaces, and seeks to regulate the spaces where disabled people are deemed to be 'at risk'. In so doing, Edwards draws on an analysis which acknowledges that both space and law are socially constructed entities, a product of social, cultural and political processes rather than value-free 'givens'. In this way disabled people, those framed as 'incapable minds' are seen to have 'regulated' and 'troublesome' sexual identities, and as victims and potential perpetrators of inappropriate sexual behaviour.

In Chapter 3, Grech responds to a number of concerns emerging from disability geographers based within the global South. Disability in the global South is often not contemplated in Western disability studies as a topic of analysis. When disability in the global South does become a subject of analytical inquiry, research discourse and strategies are transferred indiscriminately from the West to the rest. This is most clearly marked in discussions surrounding the word 'poverty' and its relationship to disability. Too often, references to southern disability poverty and disabled people's experience of it are opportunistically used as the central reference to disability in the majority world. Rarely are these considered epistemologically. Drawing from ethnographic work in rural Guatemala, Grech seeks to critically engage with dominant understandings of disability poverty by arguing that disability is constructed and lived differently within specific spaces and places of poverty. Poverty is thus spatially stratified and differentiated, imbued with local situated meanings and understandings. These are dynamic spaces where the meaning of disability is fluid and constantly re/negotiated, subverting attempts at homogenising both disability and the disability experience.

In Chapter 4 Roulstone and Morgan address the very topical issue of changing welfare policy constructions of disability and desert. To date there has been much writing about welfare and welfare-work reform, but most writings are concerned with the economic impact of reform on disabled people's lives. This chapter is concerned with the altered public climate that is engendered by wider welfare policy discourses that are actively repositioning social understandings of disability and welfare. Indeed, public space, even when considered within disability research, tends to be understood as a technical, physical measureable space external to the individual. Drawing on examples of changing public discourse, the chapter explores the space between disabled people's self-perceptions and the increasingly harsh welfare and media discourses around 'not genuinely disabled people'. In this sense enabling or disabling space is part physical, part social and part psychological transaction. The increasingly political emphasis on sifting the 'real' disabled people from the army of 'malingering opportunists' ignores the complex relationship between the individual, the environment and the economy. It also ignores medical, welfare and wider social constructions of just who counts as disabled. Disabled people can feel they are genuinely disabled in one definition and context and not another. In this chapter Roulstone and Morgan problematise space and acceptance/jeopardy to think about space as contested terrain, both imagined and real, where lives are constructed as more or less acceptable in a new corporeal (bodily) economy. The chapter suggests that this has led to a number of major jeopardies, especially for those disabled people who no longer fit stereotyped images of disability with the onset of new welfare discourses of disability and desert. Risks are mapped out which are countered through the new forms of resistance being practised by some disabled people's organisations as repertories of action to counter the new moral economy of neoliberal welfare.

Chapter 5 makes a marked conceptual turn to the previous chapters. Grover and Soldatic undertake a comparative analysis of the complex temporalities operating within Australian and UK spaces of social (in)security as the central mechanisms giving legitimacy to retracting disability welfare regimes. Like Edwards before them, Grover and Soldatic conceptualise the space of social security law as a space in and of itself that adopts a range of discursive, symbolic and material strategies to shift the boundaries of who can now legitimately count as disabled. While the analysis seeks to comparatively differentiate those local practices of reshaping disability welfare regimes at the national scale, Grover and Soldatic elucidate the ways in which disability geographers need to overcome the desire to focus solely on the spatial, at the risk of marginalising the role of the temporal in reshaping disability social security regimes. The chapter examines key departures and differences between the two nations, encouraging readers to critically engage with the local particularisms of how neoliberal restructuring affects disabled people. Spaces of affordance in welfare, who counts as eligible and the shifting of the disability category (Stone, 1984) is central to our understanding of the temporal-spatiality of these reforms.

In Chapter 6, the first chapter in part two of the book Reeve explores the limits to environmental improvements at the heart of reasonable adjustments or accommodations. As in previous chapters that have explored legal and spatial issues, Reeve notes how the law not only fails to adjust in an enabling way, but by making reasonableness a province of non-disabled designers and arbiters, may lead to negative and disabling social and psychological consequences. Although disabled people in the UK had the right to use services and access goods in 1995, it was only in 2004 that the Disability Discrimination Act (now the Equality Act 2010) was extended to demand that service providers make 'reasonable adjustments' to physical features which otherwise made it difficult for disabled people to access their services. Reeve discusses how indirect psycho-emotional disablism, a form of social oppression which impacts on emotional well-being and self-confidence, can arise from moving within 'landscapes of exclusion' (Kitchin, 1998: 351) caused by poorly thought through 'reasonable adjustments' (Titchkosky, 2012). While adjustments to the environment facilitate independence through the provision of physical access, this is often at the cost of disabled people's self-esteem and dignity. If the reasonable adjustment is too demeaning to use, then ironically the 'solution' to a physical barrier reinforces ablest practices of psycho-emotional disablism which is in some ways worse than no provision at all.

Warren and Garthwaite in Chapter 7 assert that place, space and identity are often closely intertwined. Based on their research on regional change and long-term impairment and health conditions, they ask: why do some localities have much higher incidence of impairment and chronic illness than others? They also ask: why do social policy initiatives and health interventions work in some areas and make little impact elsewhere? Warren and Garthwaite argue that critical disability studies perspectives are required in order to confront official spatial constructions of illness and disability. Their chapter argues that this will challenge the way in which public health researchers and geographers have tended to focus on composition or contextual effects of ill health, paying little or no attention to regional economic, psycho-social and generational factors in social understandings of disability and ill health (Macintyre *et al.*, 2002). They argue that it is only by situating constructions of disability, health and opportunity in spatial terms that a more integrated understanding of spaces, place, body and identity can emerge. The chapter argues that there is a need to understand places as entities with specific identities which are more than the sum of their parts, and that spaces are constituted by many more factors than geographical boundaries alone. The discussion draws on Wright Mills' (1959) ideas about the relationship between biography, history and social reality, and empirically reveals the implications of such an approach via a case study of the former mining district of Easington in County Durham, north-east England.

Chapter 8 explores a very tangible example of how spatial impacts of policy change can begin to afford greater policy choices in the lives of disabled people. Using the example of Scotland, a country which has successfully fostered devolved powers for certain policy areas, Hall notes how such devolution of governance is a powerful contemporary policy process. The chapter argues that aspirations for the reform of social care/support and growing disillusionment with English policy developments, has been central to the case for and practice of such devolution.

The chapter examines how the new scales and networks of social care policy-making have produced a model that is distinctly different to and challenges the individualised model of personalisation, so dominant in neoliberal welfare states including England. Further, the chapter argues that the 'double devolution' to the local authority scale in Scotland offers an opportunity for a more positive and progressive interpretation of the widely critiqued notion of 'localism'. The chapter sees this further local devolution as a recognition of the centrality of local contexts, networks, organisations, and disabled people and families, for the provision of ethically-informed practices and relationships of 'care' and 'caring'.

Other chapters in this book have helpfully documented the fact that disabled people are at times excluded from public spaces, resulting in many spending a disproportionate amount of their time in segregated social care and domestic settings or when in public space facing environmental and economic barriers to both 'being' and 'doing'. To begin, Hollomotz and Roulstone in Chapter 9 explore the less well-trodden territory of sexual citizenship for some disabled people, most especially those with learning difficulties (referred to as intellectual disabilities in many countries and as learning disabilities by official governmental authorities in England), by looking at denial of intimacy in group home contexts. Prior to moving on to the disabled people's lived experience of sexual citizenship within the context of group homes, Hollomotz and Roulstone first undertake a detailed, critical review of the broader literature on space, power and citizenship and show how this is related to disabled people's sexual citizenship. The latter half of the chapter then moves to explore these themes in the lives of people with learning difficulties through in-depth interviews with people with learning difficulties and focus groups with a self-advocacy group. The chapter concludes that the right to 'privacy' so that disabled people can fully explore and engage in practices of sexual citizenship must be formally acknowledged and enforced in social policy, and in enabling practices of support staff who have extensive authority over the lives of people with learning difficulties within their own homes. The chapter notes how pre-existing assumptions of learning difficulty have tended to err on the side of constructing sex and sexual choices for people with learning difficulties as secondary to protection from risk and the effects of 'innate vulnerability' (see Chapter 2 in this volume and Roulstone *et al.* in Roulstone and Mason-Bish, 2012). Sexual activity and desire for people with learning difficulties continues to be constructed as risky, deviant or asexual (O'Callaghan and Murphy, 2007).

Power's chapter, the final chapter in Part II, is concerned with the increasingly placeless but personalised nature of social support for people with learning difficulties. Drawing on empirical research in Ireland and Canada, Power's chapter makes clear the role of new professional support workers in the form of community connectors and social interpreters who have a role of linking disabled people with novel and uncliched social opportunities. Power's analysis illuminates the ways in which this is no longer fixed spatially and within institutional settings and requires a detailed and critical reflexive knowledge of communities and natural supports that could be identified in these fluid locations. Power makes clear that although there are some clear strides being made towards greater living options, the shortage of funding and often anti-statist nature of the wider policy reforms could risk stopping off choices, especially those for collective lifestyles options that many disabled people still wish to pursue (Roulstone and Morgan, 2009). However, with the right funding and a genuine ethic of choice, such facilitative professional roles could mark a clear step forward in aiding independence and choice for disabled people.

The discussions in this book make plain that although space and disability are being more carefully and critically connected as ideas, there is still some distance to travel in making those connections substantial and enduring. The spotlight on policy, its spatial role and influence is however seen as a very important development, as are robust empirical and cross-national evidence. To understand space and disability we clearly need to draw on the wide array of insights the book provides, connecting the overlapping ways in which they shape the lived experience of disability. We hope you enjoy reading the book.

References

Blomley, N K 1989, 'Text and context: rethinking the law-space nexus', *Progress in Human Geography*, vol. 13, no. 4, pp. 512–534.

Butler, R and Parr, H (eds) 1999, *Mind and body spaces: geographies of illness, impairment, and disability*, Routledge, London.

Chouinard, V, Hall, E C and Wilton, R (eds) 2010, *Towards enabling geographies: 'disabled' bodies and minds in society and space*, Ashgate, Farnham.

Crooks, V A, Chouinard, V and Wilton, R D 2008, 'Understanding, embracing, rejecting: women's negotiations of disability constructions and categorizations after becoming chronically ill', *Social Science and Medicine*, vol. 67, no. 11, pp. 1837–1846.

Gleeson, B 1999, *Geographies of disability*, Routledge, London.

Hansen, N 2002, 'Passing through other people's spaces: disabled women, geography and work', PhD thesis, University of Glasgow.

Haraway, D 1991, *Simians, cyborgs, and women: the reinvention of women*, Routledge, London and New York.

Imrie, R 1996, *Disability and the city*, Paul Chapman Press, London.

Imrie, R 2007, 'The interrelationships between building regulations and architects' practices', *Environment and Planning B: Planning and Design*, vol. 34, no. 5, pp. 925–943.

Kitchin, R M 1998, '"Out of place", "knowing one's place": space, power and the exclusion of disabled people', *Disability and Society*, vol. 13, no. 3, pp. 343–356.

Kumari-Campbell, F 2009, *Contours of ableism: the production of disability and abledness*, Palgrave Macmillan, Victoria.

Macintyre, S, Ellaway, A and Cummins, S 2002, 'Place effects on health: how can we operationalise, conceptualise and measure them?', *Social Science & Medicine*, vol. 55, pp. 125–139.

Maddern, J and Stewart, E 2010, 'Biometric geographies, mobility and disability: biologies of culpability and the biologised spaces of (post) modernity', in V Chouinard, E Hall and R Wilton (eds), *Towards enabling geographies*, Ashgate, Farnham, pp. 237–253.

O'Callaghan, A C and Murphy, G H 2004, 'Capacity of adults with intellectual disabilities to consent to sexual relationships', *Psychological Medicine*, vol. 34, no. 7, pp. 1347–1357.

O'Callaghan, A and Murphy, G H 2007, 'Sexual relationships in adults with intellectual disabilities: understanding the law', *Journal of Intellectual Disability Research*, vol. 51, no. 3, pp. 197–206.

Oliver, M and Barnes, M 2012, *The new politics of disablement*, Palgrave Macmillan, Tavistock.

Ong, A 2006, *Neoliberalism as exception: mutations in citizenship and sovereignty*, Duke University Press, Durham, NC.

Roulstone, A and Mason-Bish, H (eds) 2012, *Disability, hate crime and violence*, Routledge, London.

Roulstone, A and Morgan, H 2009, 'Neo-liberal individualism or self-directed support: are we all speaking the same language on modernising adult social care?', *Social Policy and Society*, vol 8, no. 3, pp. 333–345.

Roulstone, A and Prideaux, S 2012, *Understanding disability policy*, Policy Press, Bristol.

Stone, D 1984, *The disabled state*, Macmillan, Basingstoke.

Titchkosky, T 2012, *The question of access: disability, space and meaning*, University of Toronto Press, Toronto.

Wright Mills, C 1959, *The sociological imagination*, Oxford University Press, Oxford.

Part I
Conceptualising disability
Spaces and places of policy exclusion

1 Space, place and policy regimes

The changing contours of disability and citizenship

Rob Imrie

Introduction

> Far from my body being for me no more than a fragment of space there would
> be no space at all for me if I had no body.
>
> (Merleau-Ponty, 2002: 117)

A significant and persistent characteristic of society is disabling spaces that are
rarely sensitised to the needs of disabled people. These range from environments
that do not provide easy means of entry to buildings for people with mobility
impairments, to places that rarely consider the importance of clear, communi-
cable, signage to facilitate the navigation of people with sensory impairment
(see Emery, 2009; Saerberg, 2010). More often than not, designed environments
revolve around a spatial logic that separates people by virtue of their bodily differences and variations in cognitive and physiological capabilities. Such separa-
tions are tantamount to an infringement of disabled people's liberties, and curtail,
potentially, their rights to occupy, and to inhabit and be present in, everyday
places, the use of which is intrinsic to a person's realisation of their well-being
(Edwards, 2013; Edwards and Imrie, 2008).

Such realisation highlights the interdependence between the body and space, and
the importance of geographical relationships in shaping a person's embodiment or
their being in the world (see Merleau-Ponty, 2002; Relph, 1976). To be embodied,
as we all are, is to be emplaced spatially, and disabled people's emplacement is
crafted by disabling spatialities or encounters in/through space that reinforce the
socio-cultural marginalisation of those deemed to be impaired. The facts of such
marginalisation are well documented, and are illustrative of disabled people's lack
of power to shape their living spaces, or to redress, with any ease, manifold forms
of spatial injustice. This is characterised by a denial of access to, and occupation
of, place, by virtue of impairment, a state of social exclusion, or what Walker and
Walker (1997: 8) define as 'the denial (or non-realization) of the civil, political,
and social rights of citizenship' (see also Room, 1995).

The denial and/or non-realisation of rights to space, that is, curtailment of capacities to exercise self-determination, is intertwined with socio-legal systems that

define the parameters of citizenship, or what one's entitlements are within the context of state policy. The prevailing context is austerity that, since 2008, has revolved around a familiar menu of retrenchment of state expenditures, privatisation and deregulation, and is implicated in what the editors of this book describe as changes in 'the social relations of space and place'. In the chapter, I explore this statement and the multiple intersections between disability, austerity public policy and geography, noting the limited explication about the interrelationships between the lives of disabled people and the geographies of public policy, or the intrinsically spatialised nature of state policy regimes. I suggest that the development of interdisciplinary inquiry, between geography, social policy and disability studies, may be a basis for enhancing understanding of the impact of policy regimes on disabled people.

I divide the chapter into three parts. I begin by outlining the case for the focus on the inherently geographical nature of policy regimes in which, as I shall argue, the fortunes of disabled people have to be understood as indissoluble from the intersections between space, place and policy. Such intersections, in the context of a post-welfare world, are shaped, in part, by the human worthiness of disabled people being, increasingly, discredited in a context whereby welfare policy reform is placing the onus on self-active and self-starting individuals as the basis of a good society. I develop this discussion in the second part of the chapter where I focus on the diminution of disabled people's liberties with reference to place-based restructuring in three different policy domains in the UK, housing, transport and public space. In each instance, public policy is intersecting with place to recreate spaces of exclusion or environs that deny opportunity for selfhood.

I conclude the chapter by outlining the need to (re-)politicise the body as part of the development of what citizenship is or ought to be, in ways whereby impairment becomes regarded as the normalcy of everyday life. The assertion, of the normalcy of impairment, does, however, challenge the socio-cultural constructions of disability in society, including the crafting of disabling spatialities that render, potentially, impairment as an object of disablement. I suggest that these relations (of disablement) may be challenged by the development of a body politics that develops the discourse that everyone, irrespective of corporal form and performance, has the rights to inhabit, or to be emplaced, in ways whereby spaces are facilitative of a person's autonomy or the intrinsic value of the self.

Policy regimes, citizenship and productive bodies

This volume is part of a new wave of writings seeking to understand the interrelationships between disability, space and public policy, and to re-direct study towards the irreducible, intersectional, nature of disablement in society. Such intersections conceive of disability as a relational phenomenon, multi-dimensional in scope, and constituted through competing discourses about embodiment. The most significant is the 'body-abject' or the elision between impairment and personal deficiency, a pejorative representation of disability that medicalises and individualises the body. Social practice towards the deficient body sifts and sorts people by bodily capabilities and capacities in relation to measures of fitness to work. Such measures, while seemingly objective, are neither neutral nor benign and are the basis of moral judgments about who are worthy, rational, subjects. Those deemed to deviate from such subject-positions are targets of state interventions to correct deviancy and provide support for self-improvement.

The social practices of disablement, that constitute the basis of disabled people's citizenship, are influenced by where they take place, that is, their particular geographical or spatial contexts (Imrie and Edwards, 2007). Disablement, as a political ideology and practice towards disabled people, is not impervious to the locales or places in which disabled people lead their lives, and one of the key arguments of the book is that place matters, not only as the context of/for embodied social practice, but, more importantly, as constitutive of those very practices (Massey, 2005). The structures and possibilities of experience, that is, the shaping of one's identity, is intertwined with space, not in any essentialist way that would ask the question 'who am I?', but, rather, where the social and the spatial are conceived as indivisible, in which one's positioning in socially defined space is characterised by asking the question 'where am I?'.

The understanding of disability as a spatial phenomenon, is, however, relatively underdeveloped. Within the discipline of geography, there is a small corpus of research on the subject, characterised by its marginality at international conferences, in geographical journals and textbooks. In a major geographical textbook, published in 2011, there are no references to, or comments about, disability, despite the authors writing a chapter about the body, place and identity (Nayak and Jeffrey, 2011). This situation is more common than not. Equally, it is rare to find writings in sociological and social policy journals that consider the geographies of disability. For instance, the 2012 Disability and Society conference featured a single article by a geographer on a non-geographical theme, and few articles with a geographical or spatial focus. In the 2011 and 2012 issues of *Disability and Society*, one article, from 44 that were published, was written by a geographer.

This need not matter if there was evidence of sustained interest in, and development of, the embodied geographies of disability, or a research disposition that recognised, after Zola (1989), that impairment is intrinsic to the human condition (see also Bickenbach and Cieza, 2011). This is not so, yet, for Zola (1989), impairment is normal and omnipresent, and this fact of matter makes it incumbent on scholarship to acknowledge how impairment, as an object of disablement, is constructed in and through its socialisation in space. This point is pertinent in relation to the social model of disability that tends to present an over-socialised understanding of disability, in which space, and disabling spatialities, are rarely articulated or part of theoretical focus. Where space is broached by the social model it appears to be as a backdrop to social actions, no more than a container that has effects on the objects contained within it.

In contrast, geographers such as Doreen Massey (2005) note that the social and the spatial are mutually entwined and constitutive insofar as social relationships and processes cannot exist outside of space. For Massey (2005), the social and the spatial are constituted in and through particular place-based social structures or

16   *R. Imrie*

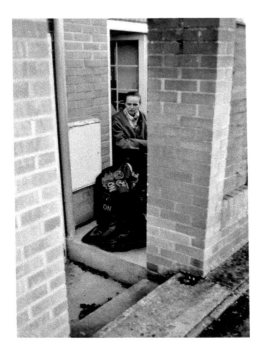

Figure 1.1 Ann, one of my research subjects from a project in the early 2000s, shows how the normal design of the dwelling does not permit her to move from the back door to the side passage where she has to deposit her weekly rubbish for collection. The design prevents her from engaging in an everyday household activity.

what she refers to as 'spatialities'. Here, space, as part of a process in the making of place, is relational, not stable or fixed, or local or bounded. Instead, it is produced and producing, imagined and materialised, structured and lived, relational, relative and absolute. Wigley (1992), drawing on De Certeau (1984), suggests that space is not a prior condition of something else but, rather, it is an outcome of part of a process of making the thing or entity we call place. In De Certeau's (1984: 117) terms, 'space is a practised place' or what Mudimbe (1991: 169) describes as 'a geography constituted by dynamic elements which meet, intersect, unite, cross each other, or diverge'.

These views point towards the need to consider what the relationship is between the role of disability in the discourse of space, and the role of space in the discourse of disability. The active, often purposive, production of bodily distinctions around disabled/abled can be identified in all facets of spatial discourse (see Gleeson, 1999; Hansen and Philo, 2007). This is evident in the physical design of any designed artefact in which there is complicity of the spatial discourse with a general, socio-cultural, subordination of impairment. Figure 1.1 shows an all too typical situation in which the space is literally producing the effect of disability (see also Edwards, 2013). It is characterised by an inequality of treatment of those whose bodies are unable to conform to the spatialities of the 'body-normal'. The outcome, disablement, is illustrative of the power of disabling design discourse as a naturalistic part of the crafting of the designed environment and, as such, it is rarely problematised or subject to critique.

The manifold nature of disabling spatialities, and their more or less taken-for-granted nature, makes it incumbent on scholarship not only to consider how impairment is manifest in space, but how space is invested with matter inimical to individuals with impairment (Freund, 2001; Gleeson, 1999; Imrie, 1996; Vellani, 2013). Such matter, from thoughtless design that prevents ease of access to places, to negative representations of disabled people that reinforce a sense of the abnormality of impairment, are intertwined with the governance of the subject, or the ways in which disabled people are defined by the state as citizens. For disabled people, their rights to be, to inhabit, or occupy space, are dependent, in part, on socio-legal principles that, through their application via state policy, are implicated in the production of disabling spaces, or spatialities that render disabled people as less than full citizens (see Vellani, 2013).

These interrelationships between geography and public policy, in the production of socio-spatial demarcations or exclusions from society, form the bedrock of written histories about disability (see Davis, 1995; Nielsen, 2012). For instance, Susan Schweik's (2010) important book, on the Ugly Laws in the United States, describes the use of local ordinances as socio-legal instruments to keep places free from the presence of particular categories of disabled people. As Schweik (2010) suggests, the laws were part of a broader societal concern with policing identities and the meaning of the body. Policing, as part of the exercise of state power, was also a feature of disabled people's incarceration into special places or locales, ranging from spaces for schooling, to asylums and dedicated work environs (see Figure 1.2). Such settings, as segregated spaces, were places for social control, to contain, and discipline, 'not normal' bodies, and to manage the presence of disabled people in everyday, mainstream, society.

While some of the more extreme versions of the state's policing of impairment have disappeared, contemporary public policy is no less likely to be implicated in disabled people's marginalisation from, and political activism in relation to, particular locales or sites of social interaction. The central thrust of this book is the understanding that, since the late twentieth century, there has been a resurgence of (neo-)liberalising government, in which experimental forms of governance, encouraging the development of post-welfare citizenship regimes, have emerged. Such regimes include the diminution of public expenditure, the retrenchment of public services, and the reduction of state interventions in the regulation of socio-institutional relations. The emphasis is one whereby citizens are required to depend less on the state for support, and to self-activate and fend for themselves by deployment of their own capabilities and resources.

This logic would have some credibility if only there was equity of capability and access to resources. For many disabled people this is not so, and their ability to cope, and influence access to life opportunities, is constrained by disabling socio-spatial formations, including the crafting of policy regimes around conceptions of

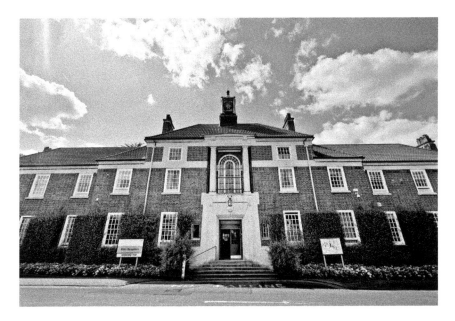

Figure 1.2 Spacing control and the governance of disability: Bethlem Royal Hospital, London.
Source: http://en.wikipedia.org/wiki/File:Bethlem_Royal_Hospital_Main_building_view_1.jpg.

corporeality that do not articulate, or recognise, the differentiated nature of bodies. Rather, neo-liberalising citizenship is premised on the undifferentiated nature of the self, or the individual defined by their relationship to market-based norms, i.e. citizenship as the exercise of individual economic agency. The difficulty for disabled people is that this instrumental logic does not equate to, or recognise, their varied and heterogeneous subject positions, or acknowledge their marginality in relation to partaking in market, exchange, relations.

The spatialisation of policy and disability

In this part of the chapter, I consider the intersections between space and policy in the lives of disabled people in the UK, and I develop the understanding that neo-liberal values are shaping the (re-)production of disabling spaces that serve to perpetuate the 'not normal' body as an aberration or a thing that resides at the margins of citizenship. These margins can be defined in terms of the relative lack of autonomy of disabled people that may suppress their sociability, or what Arendt (1958) refers to as the quality of life in civil society and civic associations. Disabled people's abilities to express autonomy is constrained and curtailed by socio-political and institutional practices that de-value particular bodily dispositions, capacities and experiences, and, consequentially, may reproduce disabling relations of dominance. This reflects the exercise of bio-power and the reduction of life to biological categories, and the subjugation of those that do not conform to socio-culturally constructed conceptions of the normal, active, body.

Public policy is powerfully entwined with discourses of/about the body, and it serves, potentially, to (re-)produce private and public realms that are not necessarily sensitive to the manifold complexities of bodies that deviate from societal norms relating to cognitive and physiological performance. This is evident in the policy field in relation to planning and spatial development, in which neo-liberal governance is to the fore (see Haughton *et al.*, 2013). Haughton *et al.* (2013: 231) refer to the dismantling of regulatory powers of state agencies responsible for spatial governance, and their supplanting by 'quasi state apparatus and indirect techniques for self-management'. For Haughton *et al.* (2013), these are the mechanisms, or techniques, of normalising 'the rationalities of neo-liberal thinking', or what they describe as the more or less inevitable ascendency of market-based forms of policy rationality.

I explore such rationalities with reference to three environs or places that are intrinsic to the crafting of a person's autonomy, and that constitute a basis for their well-being in the world. The first relates to the private realm of the home, a place that purports to provide shelter and comfort, yet functions, for many disabled people, in ways whereby their privacy and independence, or means to determine their patterns of habitation, may be denied. Such denial is intertwined with the micro-spatialities of the dwelling, and the crafting and construction of domestic spaces inattentive to impairments in ways whereby, at an extreme, there may be an inability to function, rendering a person more or less homeless. The second is transport or the means of mobility and movement in which, for many disabled people, where they can go, and at what times, is often dependent on specialised, residual, modes of mobility, such as Dial-a-Ride (DR) (for more details about DR, see Transport for London, 2013). DR, as a public service, increasingly resembles a form of post-welfare transit that serves to reinforce spatial inequalities of mobility.

The final foci are urban environments, specifically town centres that provide spaces for public interchange and interaction. Here I consider the redesign of street scapes as shared space or places that purport to create a convivial public realm that permits any user, irrespective of mode of mobility, to gain ease of access and use (see also Hamilton-Baille, 2008; Imrie, 2012). I suggest that shared space is a misnomer as its usage depends less on the provision of supportive, legible, design features to facilitate ease of navigation for all, irrespective of cognitive functioning, and more on people's individual, and uneven, sensory capacities to perceive, and make sense of, such environments. Shared spaces are a particular problem for people with sensory impairment, such as vision impaired people, and, as I argue, they are the propagation of libertarian ideas that are neither sensitised to corporeal inequalities nor supportive of those whose bodily impairment may prevent them from using, with any confidence, the designed environment.

In each instance, policy regimes, based on the market provision of goods and services, are shaping the regulation and governance of dwellings, transport and the public realm, and are constitutive of the geographies of disablement. The respective examples illustrate variations of neo-liberal policy experimentation, the outcomes of which are, potentially, the (re-)production of socially unjust spaces or places characterised by a denial of basic functioning. Such experimentation involves the fragmentation of rules, laws and, often, significant changes to regulatory environments, or what Brenner *et al.* (2009: 215) refer to as 'geoinstitutional rules regimes'. This places an onus on individuals (self-)promoting their own solutions, or, if unable to do so, becoming the subject of specialised treatment that may serve, in the case of disabled people, to be no more than a 'safety net patronage' akin to disabling forms of domination and subordination.

Market voluntarism and the death of lifetime homes

Advocates of neo-liberal policy claim it to be a harbinger of freedom by dismantling legislation and legal rules that prescribe individual conduct and courses of action (Pennington, 2006). In the UK context, the Coalition government's approach to town and country planning is an example whereby the objective is to reduce the scope of local politicians and officers in determining spatial development outcomes. Nick Boles, the planning minister, has outlined the logic whereby 'the government's feeling is that the balance between the rights of the property owner and the rights of the community could move a little further in favour of the property owner' (Ethos, 2013). To this end, the government is dismantling planning and regulatory powers to provide much more freedom to private interests to determine spatial development, and creating what Haughton *et al.* (2013) describe as soft spaces of governance (see also Allmendinger and Haughton, 2009).

Soft spaces are counterposed to the 'hard' spaces of statutory planning or regulation through formal territorial units and formal tiers of government. In contrast, the soft spaces are indicative of the de-scaling and fragmentation of formal government, and the creation of flexible institutional formations, or modes of governance to enhance the marketisation and commodification of everyday life. Soft space governance is particularly evident in relation to one of the most important locales or places that define people's lives, that is, housing. The ability to gain access to good quality housing and create a home environment invested with safety, security and personal meaning has long been a tenet of neo-conservative values (Chapman and Hockey, 1999). The home represents the bedrock of society or a place that, in its ideal sense, provides for what Chapman and Hockey (1999: 10) describe as the imaginary of 'the possibility of retreat from public view, and a place for the exercise of private dreams and fantasies'.

The reality of the home is that most people do not have control over its design or siting, and it comes pre-packaged as a thing to live in. Most dwellings are not designed with impairment in mind and lack sensitivity to the manifold ways in which bodies interact with physical objects. The recent, post-1980, history of housing policy in the UK is deregulation of government controls relating to density and space standards, and minimal regulation of internal design. The one

counter was the recognition of the needs of an ageing population, and encourage-
ment by government for the design of dwellings to enable people to age in place.
In 1999, Part M of the building regulations required builders to provide minimum
access to dwellings, and enhanced facilities, such as an accessible downstairs toilet. By the early 2000s, there was momentum for lifetime homes (LTH) standards
to become statutory for new-build housing, and some local authorities, including
the Greater London Authority, had made progress in incorporating these into planning and housing standards.[1]

The Coalition government is reversing much of this progress. Its approach to
design standards for housing reflects a shift towards voluntarism, or soft governance, by providing builders with discretion and scope to act according to their
interpretations of what the market will bear in relation to the design of dwellings.
For the government, the design of dwellings is not a matter of central dictat and is
best left to market forces or 'industry-led guidance to enable local strategic planning and delivery of this diversity of provision [for older people]' (DCLG, 2011:
49). Government policy recognises the importance of LTH to enable independent
living but says that they do 'not intend to introduce national regulation' to enforce
standards (DCLG, 2011: 49). Instead, they prefer to allow decisions about this to
be made by local authorities, sensitised to local need and in conjunction with partner organisations, including house-builders.

This appears reasonable, and laudable, until the realisation that house-builders
rarely respond to voluntary design standards or anything that is not inscribed in
legislation (see Imrie, 2006). LTH standards are slipping off the agenda and reflect
Choy's (2013: 1) characterisations of house-building design standards more generally that, since the shift from New Labour to a Coalition government, there has
been a 'transition from definitive and prescriptive statements to elective and advisory comments'. For Choy (2013), this is consistent with the neo-liberalisation of
design in permitting builders to more or less self-regulate through the contours of
soft modes of governance, as the prerequisite to enabling the diminution in building costs, and the maximisation of value or profit. Designing the micro-spaces of
the dwelling to be attentive to the body's interactions with design is unlikely to
feature as part of developers' profit/cost calculus.

Mobility, movement and post-welfare transit

While the home is important as a place to secure a person's privacy and well-
being, people's lives are also constituted by their access to social networks that
exist beyond the immediacy of the dwelling. Access is a prerequisite of sociability and the crafting of the social world, and it underpins, and shapes, how
far people can be autonomous and exercise degrees of self-determination in their
lives. Intrinsic to this is the means of mobility and movement, and here the role of
transportation is crucial in facilitating a life that enables a person to flourish as a
sociable being, or what Ben-Ishai (2008: 3) describes as 'the capacity to live one's
life according to one's own plans' (see also Arendt, 1958; Fraser, 1990). Mobility
is a prerequisite of the freedom to be, and it provides a means to be part of the

public realm, or what Beunderman *et al.* (2007: 114) define as 'a shared resource and site of exchange, interaction and collective experiences'.

In surveys of what most affects the quality of disabled people's lives, transport, and the means of mobility and movement, is paramount (Barnes, 1991). Data show that disabled people are less likely to drive private motor vehicles than non-disabled people and are, consequentially, more dependent on access to public transport (Jolly *et al.*, 2006). Such access is, however, constrained by the logic of neo-liberal policy regimes that, for Enright (2012: 797), are not 'aimed at facilitating capacities for public movement'. Rather, the development of mass transit systems is part of an economic logic to encourage investment flows and private-sector-led spatial development. Far from public transit serving a collective interest, or seeking to respond to the needs of all within residential settings, it is structured around static spatial and temporal flows to facilitate, primarily, commuter movement. This patterning is orientated towards the movement of productive bodies.

The mentalities of neo-liberalism, as evidenced in austerity and public sector retrenchment, are also changing the spatialities of mobility in places such as London, and reducing freedoms for many disabled people. The austerity drive has led the main transport provider, Transport for London (TfL), to reduce its targets for ensuring railway stations are step-free to the platform from 29 per cent to 26 per cent by 2018, and for making bus stops fully accessible from 75 per cent to 65 per cent by 2018. The numbers of underground station staff, who provide advice and support to disabled people on the network, are being cut, and pedestrian crossings in London are being eliminated, despite Transport for All (TfA, 2011: 1) noting 'that many blind people cannot cross the road without them'. It is the expectation that people will find other ways to ensure their safe movement across roads, and that they will facilitate their mobility more generally by recourse to personal, private, means.

Cuts to mainstream services are placing pressure on specialised services, such as Taxicard, Capital Call and DR, yet as TfA (2011: 1) note, funding for these 'has been frozen or cut and no plans for improving the service are mentioned'.[2] It concludes that 'in the past year, changes to door-to-door service funding have increased isolation in the capital' (TfA, 2011: 1). A rationality of market provision is taking centre stage with significant cuts to, and closures of, DR services in a range of localities around the UK. For instance, Banburyshire Community Transport Association in Oxfordshire stopped operating the county's DR service in June 2012 after two of the funders, Cherwell District Council and the County Council, reduced the budget by £220,000. In Cheshire budget cuts to DR by local councils of £165,000 has led to a reduced service and the introduction of fares (Taylor, 2013). A local councillor has commented that 'this decision on budgetary savings flies against common decency and respect' (Taylor, 2013: 1).

The neo-liberal logic of mobility means, potentially, the reduction in many disabled people's opportunities to move around, and their consignment to residual services that may reflect, and reinforce, pejorative values and attitudes of/about disability as secondary status. While DR can open up patterns of mobility for

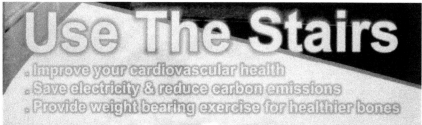

Use The Stairs

- Improve your cardiovascular health
- Save electricity & reduce carbon emissions
- Provide weight bearing exercise for healthier bones

If you feel you're very unfit start by just using the stairs to go down, if you've a long journey start by using the stairs for only part of your journey, it all helps.

Climb the stairs at normal speed	Weight in Stones 7 - 10	Weight in Stones 10 - 12	Weight in Stones 12 - 14	Weight in Stones 14 - 16
Calories burnt per minute	6.5	7.8	8.9	10

Each time you use the stairs instead of the lift you're saving electricity and carbon. The lifts in Capital House alone generate approximately 29.36 tonnes of carbon a month so if only 10% of users take the stairs instead we will save over 35 tonnes of CO_2 a year. Every little helps..

Figure 1.3 A classic piece of 'nudge'.

people who would otherwise be house-bound, access to it is premised on people meeting prescribed medical criteria relating to bodily incapacity.[3] People have to prove their incapacity to be rendered mobile by DR, to be labelled as medical subjects, a scenario that may do no more than 'blame the victim', and draw attention to individual, physiological, deficits. The irony is that in the context of the privatisation of (personal) mobility in society, including the provision of public transport to service the productive body, DR, even in a context of cutbacks, may well be the only option for many disabled people to facilitate their mobility, despite its medical overtones and reductive conception of impairment.

Libertarian paternalism and the public realm

An important part of neo-conservative agendas is the dismantling of prescriptive rules and regulations that constrain people's behaviour, hence creating contexts in which people are 'free to do what they like' (Thaler and Sunstein, 2008: 5). Thaler and Sunstein's (2008) advocating of libertarian paternalism (LP), popularly known as 'nudge theory', has gained ascendency in Coalition government policies. Corbett and Walker (2013) describe LP as deriving from a libertarian critique of the state, in which the appropriate role of government is to facilitate consumer empowerment. This is achieved less by big government legislating for change, and more by steering individuals towards behaviour commensurate with the enhancement of their welfare. Advocates of LP claim that this can be achieved

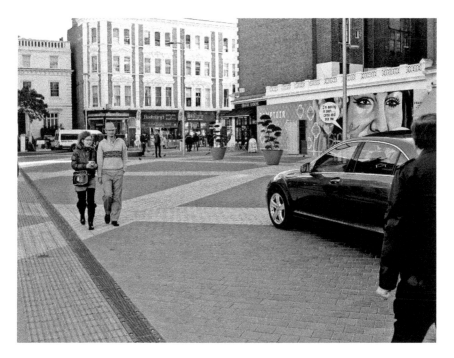

Figure 1.4 Shared space, Exhibition Road, London.

by transforming the contexts in which people make decisions about their behaviour. An example of LP in practice is the provision of information in public places about the health and personal benefits of behaviour change, such as walking to work and using stairs instead of lifts in buildings (see Figure 1.3).

The underlying idea of the message depicted in Figure 1.3 is to nudge people towards appropriate life choices instead of government legislating for changes in behaviour. This view chimes with the libertarian ideal of freeing people up to choose, unfettered by big government, although, for some, LP is no more than government at a distance. This is not, necessarily, a diminution in the roles and capacities of the state, but, rather, a realignment of state–citizen relationships that seek to place more (self-)responsibility on individuals for their actions. LP appears to have filtrated into most aspects of everyday life, and it is particularly to the fore in the design of the public realm. A popular approach, adopted by many local authorities in the UK and worldwide, is shared space, or the redesign of traditional high streets by merging pavements and roads to create a single, shared, surface (see Figure 1.4). The objective is to create calmer, safer, spaces attractive for people to visit and occupy (see Hamilton-Baille, 2008).

The advocates of shared space feel that this outcome can be achieved not by segregating users but by encouraging them to mix in the same spaces, including a mixing of bicycles, motor vehicles and pedestrians (Clarke, 2006; Hamilton-

Baille, 2008). The rationale of shared space is that no one has priority of access or usage; it is an egalitarian space. The approach is to redesign streets by removing signage or anything that signals priority of use. The logic is that such design modifications will induce cautious behaviour in users and make them more attentive to others in ways whereby everyone will feel free and able to enter such spaces without fear for their safety. It is assumed that shared space, by virtue of a redesign of town centre streets, will assure behaviour change by motorists, cyclists and others, as part of a guarantee that orderly conduct in, and enhancement of, the public realm.

Shared space is based on the deployment of positivistic, experimental knowledge about people's behaviour that does not reveal the complexities of peoples' interactions (with-)in public spaces. Most shared space schemes are not rigorously evidence based or derived from robust measures of bodily interactions with(-in) design. They are based on a design determinism in assuming (free) behaviour will follow design, or be shaped by the physical crafting of the designed environment. Human behaviour is rarely predictable and not easily absorbed into a technology such as a designed space. Rather, human behaviour and design are conjoined; they are constitutive elements in a process of becoming that is specific to the context, or the particular arrangement of people and objects in space. There is no understanding of how different bodies may interact, or perform, in different shared space environs. To all intents, it is assumed that all bodies are more or less normal, and are equal and have the capacity to enter, equally, into such spaces.

This is not so, and the conception of bodily freedom that underpins shared space design fails to recognise the unequal capacities of bodies. The particular problem of shared space is the disabling nature of its design that conceives of the citizen as an idealised individual defined by, primarily, an ocular culture, or one whereby the primacy of seeing is paramount. This is not dissimilar to Emery's (2009: 31) observation about society's perception of deaf people in which social policy is 'made in the image of hearing culture'. This holds too for shared space in which to enter into, and make sense of, such spaces require a sensory dexterity that assumes the existence of the fully functional, multisensory, subject. Shared space environments are no-go areas for vision impaired people, and part of a remake of urban space that places primacy of aesthetics over functionality in a context whereby the major motive for street redesign is to enhance the commercial viability of the public realm (for an extended discussion of these arguments, see Imrie, 2012, 2013).

Conclusion

Harvey (2008: 38) observes that the right to the city is increasingly the preserve of private interests, characterised by elite groups controlling who can gain access to, and consume, different parts of the urban environment. Public policy is entwined with the (re-)production of elite spaces, or places that reflect the primacy of market values, and the commodification of the public realm. Such commodification extends to the valuation of the body, and the interplay between bodily aesthetics, corporeal performance and processes of inclusion or exclusion from public goods, services and spaces. The embodied nature of the consumer, for consumer is what people are regarded as, is based on a reductive understanding of the body that fails to recognise, in any significant sense, corporeal complexity and the omnipresence of impairment in society. Spaces, and the places that ensue, are vested with disabling values, and shaped by processes of disablement that, far from freeing up disabled people, require them to conform in ways that constrain rather than enable them.

This feels a long way from liberal ideals of freedom and, for many disabled people, being required to 'self-activate', and take responsibility for the limitations imposed by impairment is the reality of emergent neo-liberalising policy regimes. From housing to transport and urban public space, policy reflects a (re-)conceptualisation of the citizen that is shifting from what Kumar (2012: 363) describes as collective-based understandings of citizenship to more individual ones. This revolves around the marketisation of everyday life, in which the facilitation of freedom requires one to gain access to, and participate in, the market, while, simultaneously, freeing oneself from the shackles of the state. The difficulty for many disabled people is at least twofold, one, that their participation in markets requires a 'market presence', including access to jobs, money and resources, which many do not have, and, two, in a world where impaired bodies are devalued, or non-recognised, it is unclear how disabled people can be rendered 'free'.

This is compounded by the embedded nature of disabling discourse that fails to recognise the intrinsic nature of impairment in society, and that operates with a reductive logic that measures bodily capacity, hence capability, through the lens of economic criteria, such as performance, productivity and efficiency. The elision between impairment and pejorative representations of the body, relating to lack of capacity, inefficiency and non-productivity, is part of socio-cultural conditioning of/about corporeality that constrains the nature of market provision or, at least, does not encourage responsiveness to the needs of disabled people. For many providers of goods and services, disability is an irrelevant category, and disabled people do not, in their views, constitute the basis of/for a market. It is rare to find, for instance, house-builders that have knowledge of impairment, or are likely to design a dwelling to incorporate the micro-designed features to enable ease of use by people with different types of mobility and sensory impairments.

This returns to the focus of the chapter, and the book, that is, disabling spatialities and the role of policy regimes in the (re-)production of disablism in society. Why is disabling discourse with(-in) spatial practice so resistant to change? In spatial practice, such as architecture and planning, disability is underpinned by a spatial logic of separation that is rarely a focus of a body politics or a progressive politics of well-being. For Lefebvre (1991), and others, the consequential socio-spatial marginality of particular groups, such as disabled people, needs to be described, documented and politicised as part of the rights of citizens to exercise autonomy, and to be empowered not only to imagine the possibilities of alternative, counter-mainstream, spatialities, but to enact them by being able to access, and influence, the means by which spatial relations are conceived, conceptualised and translated into place-based experiences.

The realisability of a radical politics of space, in which impairment and a critique of disabling spatialities is at its heart, is not easily achievable, yet is core to the task of creating a non-disabling society. Despite much research about disability and impairment, we are still at formative stages in understanding the complexities of disabling socio-spatial formations. There are some instructive works for guidance, including Emery (2009) who outlines how Deaf communities draw attention to the phonocentric nature of citizenship that assumes that hearing is normal. In doing so, they highlight how spaces are socially constructed around 'hearing places' that exclude those that do not hear. Likewise, vision impaired groups have described, in the case of shared space, and other places, the dominance of visuality in shaping spatial relations (Guide Dogs for the Blind Association, 2006). Documentation of such experiences is important to show how impairment interacts with(-in) socially constructed spaces as part of disablement in society.

In and of itself, such documentation of hegemonic spaces, and their crafting around the 'body normal', is insufficient, and a politics of disablement must, simultaneously, be a politics of space that has regard to the different ways in which disablism is manifest in and through place. This politics is necessarily one of resistance to hegemonic conceptions, representations and categories of/about disability and the body, and will assert the normalcy of impairment, or the body as a dynamic and transient subject, never fixed nor stable.

Acknowledgement

My thanks to Sarah Fielder who read a draft of the chapter and provided insights that enabled me to clarify key arguments.

Notes

1 Lifetime homes (LTH) are operated by the Habinteg Housing Association, and have their origins in the 1990s. Habinteg describe them on its website as 'a set of 16 design criteria that provide a model for building accessible and adaptable homes'. Principle 8, for instance, says that 'An entrance level living room provides an accessible space to socialise with the household for any visitor regardless of their level of mobility'. Such standards seek to ensure that for mobility impaired people, new housing can be easily accessed and used and is designed in ways to facilitate ageing in place through the life course. LTH have been written into the London Plan that requires all new homes within the Greater London Authority to meet the standard. For further details see: www.lifetimehomes.org.uk/pages/lifetime-homes-design-guide.html, accessed 19 June 2013.

2 Such specialised services are notorious for their unreliability and lack of flexibility in responding to individual needs. Brown and Harris (2009: 17) report findings from a study of DR in Barnet, North London: 'Dial-a-Ride was a mode of transport that was useful but not always reliable. They did not always "show up", it is "not as good as they could be", but it is "free". It was reported that changes to the booking system for Dial-a-Ride had meant that block-bookings to take groups of people were not possible and three separate Dial-a-Ride mini vans could arrive at a day centre to pick up three people simultaneously.'

3 The medicalised qualification process includes a range of criteria, including: to be in receipt of the Higher Rate Mobility Component of the Disability Living Allowance; to be registered blind; to be in receipt of Higher Rate Attendance Allowance (for women aged over 60 and men aged over 65); and, to be in receipt of the Mobility Supplement of the War Pension (see Brown and Harris, 2009).

References

Allmendinger, P and Haughton, G 2009, 'Soft spaces, fuzzy boundaries and metagovernance: the new spatial planning in the Thames Gateway', *Environment and Planning A*, vol. 41, pp. 617–633.

Arendt, H 1958, *The human condition*, Chicago University Press, Chicago.

Barnes, C 1991, *Disabled people in Britain and discrimination*, Hurst and Company, London.

Ben-Ishai, E 2008, 'The autonomy-fostering state: citizenship and social service delivery', PhD thesis, University of Michigan.

Beunderman, J, Hannon, C and Bradwell, P 2007, *Seen and heard: reclaiming the public realm with children and young people*, DEMOS, London.

Bickenbach, J and Cieza, A 2011, 'The prospects for universal disability law and social policy', *Journal of Accessibility and Design for All*, vol. 1, no. 1, pp. 23–37.

Brenner, N, Peck, J and Theodore, N 2009, 'Variegated neoliberalization: geographies, modalities, pathways', *Global Networks*, vol. 10, no. 2, pp. 182–222.

Brown, K and Harris, A 2009, *The voice of experience: the unmet needs of older people in Barnet*, Age Concern, Barnet.

Chapman, T and Hockey, J (eds) 1999, *Ideal homes? Social change and domestic life*, Routledge, London.

Choy, N 2013, 'The many lives of Building for Life: design standards and the governance of housing quality', unpublished paper, available from Nicholas Choy, Department of Geography, King's College London, Strand, London, WC2R 3LS.

Clarke, E 2006, 'Shared space: the alternative approach to calming traffic', *Traffic Engineering Control*, 47(8), pp. 290–292.

Corbett, S and Walker, A 2013, 'The big society: rediscovery of "the social" or rhetorical fig-leaf for neo-liberalism?', *Critical Social Policy*, vol. 33, no. 3, pp. 451–472.

Davis, L 1995, *Enforcing normalcy: disability, deafness and the body*, Verso, London.

De Certeau, M 1984, *The practice of everyday life*, University of California Press, Berkeley.

Department of Communities and Local Government (DCLG) 2011, *Laying the foundations: a housing strategy for England*, The Stationery Office, London.

Edwards, C 2013, 'The anomalous wellbeing of disabled people: a response', *Topoi: An International Review of Philosophy*, vol. 32, no. 2, pp. 189–196.

Edwards, C and Imrie, R 2008, 'Disability and the implications of the wellbeing agenda: some reflections from the United Kingdom', *Journal of Social Policy*, vol. 37, no. 3, pp. 337–355.

Emery, S 2009, 'In space no one can see you waving your hands: making citizenship meaningful to Deaf worlds', *Citizenship Studies*, vol. 13, no. 1, pp. 31–44.

Enright, T 2012, 'Mass transportation in the neo-liberal city: the mobilizing of myths of the Grand Paris Express', *Environment and Planning A*, vol. 45, pp. 797–813.

Ethos 2013, Interview with Nick Boles MP, March, accessed 19 June 2013, www.ethosjournal.com/topics/politics/item/425-interview-with-nick-boles-mp.

Fraser, N 1990, 'Rethinking the public sphere: a contribution to the critique of actually existing democracy', *Social Text*, no. 25/26, pp. 56–80.

Freund, P 2001, 'Bodies, disability and spaces: the social model and disabling spatial organizations', *Disability and Society*, vol. 16, no. 5, pp. 689–706.

Gleeson, B 1999, *Geographies of disability*, Routledge, London.

Guide Dogs for the Blind Association 2006, *Shared surface street design research project*, Reading, The Guide Dogs for the Blind Association.

Hamilton-Baille, B 2008, 'Towards shared space', *Urban Design International*, vol. 13, pp. 130–138.

Hansen, N and Philo, C 2007, 'The normality of doing things differently: bodies, spaces and disability geography', *Tijdschrift voor economische en sociale geografie*, vol. 98, no. 4, pp. 493–506.

Harvey, D 2008, 'The right to the city', *New Left Review*, vol. 53, pp. 23–40.

Haughton, G, Allmendinger, P and Oosterlynck, S 2013, 'Spaces of neoliberal experimentation: soft spaces, postpolitics and neoliberal governmentality', *Environment and Planning A*, vol. 45, no. 1, pp. 217–234.

Imrie, R 1996, *Disability and the city*, Sage, London.

Imrie, R 2006, *Accessible housing: quality, disability, and design*, Routledge, London.

Imrie, R 2012, '"Auto-disabilities": the case of shared space environments', *Environment and Planning A*, vol. 44, no. 9, pp. 2260–2277.

Imrie, R 2013, 'Shared space and the post-politics of environmental change', *Urban Studies*, vol. 50, no. 16, pp. 3446–3462.

Imrie, R and Edwards, C 2007, 'The geographies of disability: reflections on the development of a sub-discipline', *Geography Compass*, vol. 1, no. 3, pp. 623–640.

Jolly, D, Priestly, M and Matthews, B 2006, *Secondary analysis of existing data on disabled people's use and experiences of public transport in Great Britain*, a research report for the Disability Rights Commission, DRC, London.

Kumar, A 2012, 'Educating the (neo liberal) citizen: reflections from India', *Development in Practice*, vol. 22, no. 3, pp. 361–372.

Lefebvre, H 1991, *The production of space*, Blackwell, Oxford.

Massey, D 2005, *For space*, Sage, London.

Merleau-Ponty, M 2002, *Phenomenology of perception*, Routledge, London.

Mudimbe, V 1991, *Parables and fables: exegesis, textuality and politics in Central Africa*, University of Wisconsin Press, Madison.

Nayak, A and Jeffrey, A 2011, *Geographical thought: an introduction to ideas in human geography*, Prentice Hall, London.

Nielsen, K 2012, *A disability history of the United States*, Beacon Press, Boston.

Pennington, M 2006, 'Sustainable development and British land use planning: a Hayekian perspective', *Town Planning Review*, vol. 77, no. 1, pp. 75–97.

Relph, E 1976, *Place and placelessness*, Pion, London.

Room, G 1995, *Beyond the threshold: the measurement and analysis of social exclusion*, Polity Press, Bristol.

Saerberg, S 2010, '"Just go straight ahead": how blind and sighted pedestrians negotiate space', *The Senses and Society*, vol. 5, no. 3, pp. 364–381.

Schweik, S 2010, *The ugly laws: disability in public*, New York University Press, New York.

Taylor, M 2013, 'Winsford anger grows at Cheshire West's Dial a Ride decision', *Winsford Guardian*, 17 June.

Thaler, R and Sunstein, C 2008, *Nudge: improving decisions about health, wealth, and happiness*, Yale University Press, New Haven.

Transport for All (TfA) 2011, 'Our message to the Mayor: progress on accessibility has stalled', accessed 19 June 2013, www.transportforall.org.uk/news/our-message-to-the-mayor-progress-on-accessibility-has-stalled.

Transport for London, (2013), Your Guide to Dial a Ride, London, TfL.

Vellani, F 2013, *Understanding disability discrimination law through geography*, Ashgate, Farnham.

Walker, A and Walker, C (eds) 1997, *Britain divided: the growth of social exclusion in the 1980's and 1990's*, Child Poverty Action Group, London.

Wigley, M 1992, 'Untitled: the house of gender', in B Colomina (ed.), *Sexuality and space*, Princeton University Press, New York, pp. 327–389.

Zola, I 1989 'Towards the necessary universalising of a disability policy', *The Milbank Quarterly*, vol. 67, no. 2, pp. 401–428.

2 Emplacing disabled bodies/ minds in criminal law

Regulating sex and sexual consent in Ireland's Criminal Law (Sexual Offences) Act 1993

Claire Edwards

Introduction

> The body is our vehicle for traversing space and for responding to the world's sensory stimuli; it is the location of our psyche, with its drives both creative and destructive; it is the tool we hone in order to communicate, to love and to hate; it offers a 'surface', inscribed by us and read by others; it is a sexed organism that matures, may well become diseased or maimed, and eventually dies; it is a social being on which institutions leave their imprint and by which they in turn are modified; and which is variously endowed with attributes inherent and acquired (wealth, power and so on).
>
> (Teather 1999: 12)

Understanding the complex entity that is 'the body' and the way in which bodies interact with space and place has become a key part of the geographical enterprise. As Teather's definition above suggests, the body is far more than a physical, biological entity: it forms a site for the inscription of particular values and the creation of identities, and inescapably shapes how we experience our lives, including how we interact with different spaces. Geographers concerned with exploring dimensions of disabled people's lives have particularly drawn attention to this symbiotic relationship between the body and space. Analyses have highlighted how the disabled body as a space in its own right is often devalued and stigmatised (see, for example, Edwards and Imrie 2003; Longhurst 2010), but also how the corporeal experience of impairment affects the ways in which disabled people interact with, and are sometimes excluded from, particular spaces (Parr 2008).

The embodied geographies of disabled people's everyday lives draw attention to the way in which particular institutions – from medicine to the law – have sought to regulate the disabled body and its associated habits and behaviours as a way of maintaining and managing societal norms. The history of disability in the Western world has been one in which the creation of special institutions and welfare programmes and policies 'have created, classified, codified, managed and controlled anomalies through which some people have been divided from others and objectivised as (for instance) physically impaired, insane, handicapped, mentally ill, retarded, and deaf' (Tremain 2005: 6). This process of classifying has had consequences for the types of spaces society deems it 'legitimate' for disabled people to occupy, and how disabled people themselves negotiate and seek to reclaim spaces which are premised on ableist values and norms (Chouinard 1999; Dyck 2010).

In this chapter, I deploy these ideas to explore a debate taking place in Ireland in 2013 concerning people with intellectual disabilities' right to a sexual relationship. In particular, I focus on the ongoing review by the State's Law Reform Commission of a piece of legislation, Section 5 of the Criminal Law (Sexual Offences) Act 1993 which in seeking to protect people with intellectual disabilities from sexual abuse, also makes it unlawful for two people with intellectual disabilities to have a consenting sexual relationship unless they are married. People with intellectual disabilities represent a group for whom ideas of sexuality have been, and frequently still are, subject to contention and negativity. Societal perceptions have often swung between viewing people with intellectual disabilities as child-like beings with no sexual desires, to constructing them as sexually threatening (Block 2000; Hollomotz 2009). In Ireland, the uncertainty in terms of how best to respond to the sexual desires of people with intellectual disabilities has become obvious in public attitude surveys towards disability: a recent study found that respondents were less likely to support the idea of people with intellectual disabilities having a right to a sexual relationship compared to other impairment groups (such as people with physical or sensory impairments) (National Disability Authority 2011). The main reasons given for this were the lack of capacity of people with intellectual disabilities to make decisions or give consent.

The review of Section 5 taking place in Ireland draws particular attention to how law, as both an institution and set of procedures, is implicated in subjugating the bodies/minds[1] of people with intellectual disabilities, and regulating their interaction with different types of space. As scholars within the sub-discipline of 'critical legal geographies' have shown, law is intimately intertwined with socio-spatial relations, shaping how particular groups or individuals use or experience space, and setting up boundaries between different groups of citizens and spaces (criminal/non-criminal, victim/offender, public/private) (Blomley 1989; Chouinard 1994). Arguably, one of the consequences of Section 5 is that it takes away any notion of private space for people with intellectual disabilities: all (sexual) relations must be subject to public scrutiny or regulation. At the same time, however, by recognising that people with intellectual disabilities can have sexual relationships if they are married, the legislation also fails to recognise how the 'private' domain can also become a site of threat, as feminist researchers have shown in the context of domestic violence (Suk 2006). Within these spaces, the values and identities ascribed to people with intellectual disabilities are made and remade: by default, Section 5 has the potential to render a person with intellectual disabilities an offender or a victim in different circumstances. In exploring the 'law-space nexus' (Blomley 1989) in the context of the Criminal Law (Sexual Offences) Act 1993, then, I develop an analysis that acknowledges that both space and law are socially constructed entities: a product of social, cultural and political processes rather than value-free 'givens' as many critical legal scholars suggest (see for example Blomley and Bakan 1992; Butler 2009; Delaney *et al.* 2001).

The chapter is structured around four sections. I start by exploring the interconnections between ideas emerging from critical legal geographies and geographies of disability in trying to unpick the way in which law seeks to regulate the embodied lives of people with intellectual disabilities in relation to their sexuality. After providing a context to the emergence of the Criminal Law (Sexual Offences) Act 1993 in Ireland, I then go on to explore some of the ways in which Section 5 *emplaces* people with intellectual disabilities in criminal law. My use of the term 'emplacing' borrows from the language of human geographers who have been concerned to explore the multiple ways in which space and place play a role in constituting experiences and knowledge (see, for example, Longhurst 2001; Morin and Berg 1999). From this perspective, space is intimately tied up with shaping socio-political relations, whilst socio-political relations also give shape to space in a constantly recursive relationship. Emplacing raises questions about how the particularities of specific places or different spatial contexts (cities, localities, regions, nations and so on) give rise to different types of (bodily) knowledge or experience. In the context of this chapter, therefore, to talk of 'emplacing' disabled bodies/minds is to focus on exploring how space makes a difference to the constitution of the intellectually disabled body/mind in relation to sexuality: how, for example, do the legal systems of different places contribute to constituting this relation and identity? Or, on a micro-scale, how do people with intellectual disabilities experience their bodies in different places or types of space in terms of their sexuality (and indeed, *create* space through that experience)?

My analysis of emplacing in this chapter takes two forms. In the first instance, I explore how the bodies/minds of people with intellectual disabilities *as sites in themselves* – or as Adrienne Rich (1986: 212) famously referred to the body – 'the geography closest in' (see also Johnston and Longhurst 2010) – become inscribed with particular (moral) values. I then go on to examine how the inscription of these values has implications for the types of spaces that the intellectually disabled body/mind is deemed able to occupy in the context of debates about sexuality, and how the legislation engages in a form of boundary work to demarcate spaces of risk where people with intellectual disabilities are necessarily seen as 'out of place'. I conclude by discussing the further potential of geographical work which recognises the complex interactions between disabled bodies/minds, law and space.

Situating disabled bodies/minds in law and space

In recent years, there has been a growing consciousness within the discipline of geography of the embodied experience of impairment. From its emergence as a sub-discipline over a decade ago, 'geographies of disability' focused attention on the way in which disability, in and of itself, was a socio-spatial construct, and how particular environments shaped by 'ableist' values served to exclude disabled people from society, marking them out as different in particular spaces whilst simultaneously rendering them invisible (Chouinard *et al.* 2010; Imrie and Edwards 2007; Parr 2008). The more recent shift to engage with the materiality of impairment is reflective of a growing awareness within geography and the social sciences more generally of the body/mind as both a biological and social entity, and its complex relationship with society and space. Bodies have been identified as spaces in their own right, but also as a vehicle through which we perceive the world around us, and to which other people react. Studies such as Moss and Dyck's (2002) account of the everyday geographies of women with chronic illness, or Parr's (2008) exploration of the embodied performances of people with mental illness in public spaces, shed light on the complex intertwining of the body/mind as a material and discursive entity: that is, how certain values, norms and expectations become written upon disabled bodies/minds and impact on their interaction with different environments. In so doing, these studies build on calls from within certain quarters of disability studies to 'bring the body back in' to disability theorising, as a way of bridging the perceived dualism between impairment as a biological entity and disability as a form of social oppression (Hall 2000; Hughes and Paterson 1997).

The increasing focus on the body has also resulted from the dismantling of divisions which existed in Western knowledge around the mind–body dualism. Feminist analyses have shown how the premising of mind and reason over the body was a profoundly gendered (and it should be said, racialised) activity, such that masculinity became associated with reason and rationality, and femininity with (disorderly) bodies and emotions.[2] Indeed, as Longhurst (1997: 491) notes:

> In western culture, while white men may have presumed that they could transcend their embodiment (or at least have their bodily needs met by others) by seeing it as little more than a container for the pure consciousness it held inside, this was not allowed for women, blacks, homosexuals, people with disabilities, the elderly, children and so on.

In this context, women were represented as little more than their bodies. The same might also be said of disabled people, who have often been constructed predominantly in terms of bodily and/or cognitive impairment – which in turn has allowed society to intervene and regulate the perceived risks or vulnerabilities associated with impairment. In their exploration of social policy in Australia, Bacchi and Beasley (2002) note this distinction by distinguishing between policy which frames people as having control over their bodies (and therefore not requiring state intrusion or regulation) and those who are *controlled by* their bodies. For the latter group, the lack of autonomy over their bodies signals a need for state intervention, as they are constituted as 'lesser citizens' (p. 325).

For the purposes of this chapter, it is significant to note that such interventions also become expressed spatially: for example, Parr's (2008) account of the geographies of people with mental illness charts the shift from 'carcereal geographies', where institutionalisation spatially segregated people with mental health problems, to one in which people with mental illness are seeking to challenge the disciplining tendencies of the asylum in non-institutional spaces. In these contexts, the micro-interactions of everyday geographies become apparent as particular behaviours marking people out as 'Other' are played out in public spaces and encounters. This is not just the case for people with mental illness; for example, Longhurst's (1999: 79) study of pregnant women illustrates how certain bodily forms attract (unwanted) attention and advice in public space, as well as forms of regulation. As she states, dominant ideas that associate pregnancy with emotionality and erratic behaviour act to 'disqualify them from stepping "objectively" and "dispassionately" into the public sphere long associated with "Rational Man"'. Pregnant women and their bodies become seen as a 'condition', and are thereby treated as such (see also Lupton 2012).

Studies of the embodied geographies of everyday life then expose the biological essentialism behind societal approaches and attitudes towards impairment, and how the body/mind is itself implicated in social relations. They also expose the way in which particular institutions and practices put their mark upon the body/mind. In this chapter, my particular concern is with law as a mechanism through which disabled people's lives are shaped and regulated, and which emplaces disabled people in society in multiple, and often contradictory, ways (Chouinard 1994). Law brings into being particular legal subjectivities, and sets up boundaries between different subject identities and bodies (the victim/offender; citizen/non-citizen and so on). In so doing, as critical legal geographers have shown, it also constructs and demarcates particular spaces (private and public, for example) where behaviours are deemed appropriate or inappropriate (Blomley and Bakan 1992; Delaney *et al.* 2001). Law, then, has a spatial inflection: it both constitutes space but is also transformed through it. For critical legal geographers, examining the interaction between law and space is a task that involves recognising law as a situated set of practices rather than a neutral, value-free entity as many legal scholars and, indeed, the justice system, would have us believe (Berti 2010; Butler 2009; Mitchell 2001).

This situatedness is something that feminist scholars of law in particular have drawn attention to. In discussing how law reflects the inherent values of the society within which it is located, Smart (1989) notes how perceptions about notions of femininity and appropriate behaviour come into play in rape case trials. These discourses also have a spatial component, as Sanger (2001: 31) describes in her discussion about the relationship between women and cars. In asking the question 'How does the law comprehend, affect, reinforce, transform and undermine the relations between persons and things?', she describes how the car as a space has become implicated in women's subordination by being associated with a site of sex, and hence of danger. As she states:

> The danger of riding in cars combines both physical and legal harms. Cars are dangerous not because women get raped in them, but also because accepting a ride in a man's car or offering to give a man a ride in her own car is often taken as a proxy for consent to sex.
>
> (Sanger 2001: 37)

The law, and legal judgments, frequently reinforce these gendered notions of space, often viewing the private realm of the car as an exception to the legal regulation of sexual behaviour in public spaces in cases of rape or sexual assault.

In the case of people with intellectual disabilities and the thorny issue of sexual relationships, we might also argue that the law has reinforced ableist notions of space, and inscribed particular identities which seek to keep them 'out of place' as far as sex is concerned. As several commentators have pointed out, the status of people with intellectual disabilities as sexual beings was intimately tied up with attempts in Western industrialised nations to regulate and discipline the body politic and, in particular, seek to control those elements of the population that potentially posed a social threat (Gill 2010; McDonnell 2007; Shildrick 2007a; Tremain 2005; Walmsley 2000). Walmsley (2000) for example, examines how the introduction of the Mental Deficiency Act 1913 in the United Kingdom, which enabled authorities to identify and deal with 'mental defectives', including those deemed to be 'feeble-minded', was in large part a response to try and control the sexual behaviour of women with intellectual disabilities who were seen as lacking self-control, and who, through their sexual activity and procreation, were contributing to the degeneracy of the population. Concerns about people with intellectual disabilities' sexual status often led to their institutionalisation, and in some cases, enforced sterilisation (and in many landscapes, this has remained an ongoing practice). Whilst attitudes may have shifted somewhat over the course of the twentieth century, there is still little doubt that attitudes towards people with intellectual disabilities as sexual beings are often contested and contradictory, leading them (and particularly women) to be seen as either sexually promiscuous or asexual (Hollomotz 2009; Shildrick 2007a, 2007b).This is part of a broader societal response to disability and sexuality which is frequently represented through discourses of anxiety and disgust, thereby raising questions about 'who is to count as a sexual subject' (Shildrick 2007b: 221).

One of the difficulties which legislation and other policies and procedures have struggled to address is the issue of assessing capacity to consent to sexual relationships (Gill 2010). Research has shown that people with intellectual disabilities are far more likely to be victims of sexual abuse, and sexual exploitation is a key concern (McCarthy and Thompson 1996; Sobsey 1994). To that end, legislation which exists around capacity to consent has frequently focused on protection from risk, rather than finding freedom of sexual expression. Meanwhile, the taboos that still exist around disability and sexual relationships often lead to people with intellectual disabilities not having access to appropriate sex education; Cristian *et al.* (2001: 283) also note that 'gender identity and body image may play a large part in impeding the sexual expression of women with developmental disabilities'. Part of the difficulty for many people with intellectual disabilities is that what is an activity of the private sphere becomes one of public regulation and scrutiny: the spaces of institutions, in which so many people with intellectual disabilities historically lived, are not places where sexual expression can be explored or fulfilled. Rather, they can be places where such interactions are closed down or are a source of reprimand (Kelly *et al.* 2009). In the sections that follow, I go on to explore some of these dilemmas by focussing on Ireland's Criminal Law (Sexual Offences) Act 1993 as an incidence of the spatialisation of bodily capacities in law's ordering of sexuality.

Regulating sexual consent in Irish criminal law: emplacing people with intellectual disabilities

Like many other Western nations, Ireland has a long history of the institutionalisation and segregation of people with intellectual disabilities. Concerns about managing unruly populations were a key part of Britain's colonial project in Ireland: after independence in 1922, segregationist tendencies continued through the combined rule of the Catholic Church and State which played a key role in regulating the moral and reproductive compass of the population. Eugenic concerns to control the spread of 'feeble-mindedness' manifested themselves predominantly through large scale incarceration rather than through sterilisation, which many in the Catholic Church were opposed to. As McDonnell (2007: 142) notes, however, this opposition 'was more of a defence of Catholic moral teaching than a concern for the human and civil rights of disabled people'.

Like other common law countries, Ireland introduced specific legislative provisions to protect people with intellectual disabilities from sexual exploitation. The first attempt at this was embodied in the Criminal Law Amendment Act of 1935 which sought to protect women deemed to be 'feeble-minded' from sexual intercourse (but not other forms of sexual assault or harassment). Section 4 of the Act stated:

> Any person who, in circumstances which do not amount to rape, unlawfully and carnally knows or attempts to have unlawful carnal knowledge of any woman or girl who is an idiot, or an imbecile, or is feeble-minded shall, if the circumstances prove that such person knew at the time of such knowledge or attempt that such woman or girl was then an idiot or an imbecile or feeble-minded (as the case may be), be guilty of a misdemeanour and shall be liable on conviction thereof to imprisonment for any term not exceeding two years.
>
> (Government of Ireland 1935)

The language used reflected the perceptions of the time regarding people with intellectual disabilities as abnormal and deficient: it also embodied gendered assumptions that sexual assault was only something that could be perpetrated against women. However, it was only in 1993 following a legislative review by the State's Law Reform Commission in 1990 (Law Reform Commission 1990) that this section was replaced with Section 5 of the Criminal Law (Sexual Offences) Act 1993, which exists to this date.

Section 5 states that:

> a person who – (a) has or attempts to have sexual intercourse, or (b) commits or attempts to commit an act of buggery, with a person who is mentally

impaired (other than a person to whom he is married or to whom he believes with reasonable cause he is married) shall be guilty of an offence.

(Government of Ireland 1993)

The problems with the section have been widely acknowledged, not least in the Law Reform Commission's recent consultation paper on the legislation. First, it draws on understandings of disability which are outmoded and at odds with the disability rights agenda; second, because the section does not allow for consent as a defence for a sexual relationship outside of marriage between two adults with intellectual disabilities who were both capable of consenting, it has the unintended effect of making it a criminal offence for two people with intellectual disabilities to have a sexual relationship outside marriage. Third, the Act does not protect people with 'mental impairment' against other forms of unwanted sexual behaviour and harassment, only intercourse. Fourth, it has been argued that using the notion of 'incapable of living an independent life' is not an appropriate way to assess an individual's capacity to consent to sexual relations (someone may not live fully independently but still have capacity to give consent) (Kelly *et al.* 2009). The difficulties with the Act are multiple therefore, and it is unsurprising that the Law Reform Commission in its consultation paper has proposed repealing Section 5. However, as I go on to demonstrate, the legislation says much about the way in which (Irish) society has sought to protect and regulate the bodies/minds of people with intellectual disabilities in the most intimate areas of their life, despite an emergent disability rights agenda in the State over the past 20 years which has been vehemently advocating for the equal status of people with disabilities as citizens.

Creating 'incapable' bodies and minds

One of the key contributions that have been made by theorisations of the body since the mid 1990s is a recognition that our bodies are not just 'given', but are intimately tied up in social and political relations. Whilst the range of approaches to understanding the body has been described as 'bewildering' (Edwards and Imrie 2003: 240), from Bourdieu's notion of the body as a bearer of value and social and cultural capital, to the body as a discursive site or text, it has become apparent that bodies represent neither just biology, nor society, but an intricate intertwining of the two: social values and understandings have the potential to construct and respond to biology in particular ways, and vice versa. As feminists have shown, for example, discourses of the biological body have been used to reinforce patriarchal distinctions between men and women's social status, by representing social differences in 'natural', biological terms (Bordo 1993; Longhurst 1997). Meanwhile, societal valuations which proscribe the 'perfect body' also have material consequences as people seek to work on their bodies – through exercise, dieting or, more drastically, cosmetic surgery – in an attempt to realise corporeal norms (Hall 2000).

The body as a site of interaction between biology and societal judgments becomes readily visible in the way in which Section 5 of the Criminal Law

(Sexual Offences) Act 1993 construes people with intellectual disabilities. In the first instance, it is clear that the Act views people with intellectual disabilities as (intellectually) incapable as far as sexual relationships are concerned and constructs them wholly in terms of impairment and incapacity. Mental impairment in the Act is defined as 'suffering from a disorder of the mind, whether through mental handicap or mental illness, which is of such a nature or degree as to render a person incapable of living an independent life or of guarding against serious exploitation' (Government of Ireland 1993). This is a definition strongly rooted in notions of cognitive deficit, reflecting broader societal perceptions which ground disability in the individual, in biology, and as a state which is somehow other than normal.

Indeed, in the same way that Longhurst (1997) notes how women are often constructed in terms of the messiness and unpredictability of the female body, so the bodies/minds of people with intellectual disabilities are seen as uncontrollable in relation to sex, as risky and, in some circumstances, dangerous (not least in a situation where two people with intellectual disabilities are ascribed 'offender' subjectivities if they engage in sex outside of marriage). In this context, the mind, which is seen as faulty and irrational, becomes part and parcel of the problematisation of the body; sex is perceived as an act which is somehow deviant and 'unnatural' for people with intellectual disabilities, as if in some way their bodies (and minds) were not made to engage in sexual intercourse, or at least, not engage in it within the boundaries of what is considered 'normal' sexual practice (Shildrick 2007a). The Act therefore objectifies the body, and uses biology as a way of marking out people with intellectual disabilities as different and less than human in the arena of sexuality.

One of the key difficulties of the Act is the way in which it fails to provide any definition of what consent or capacity might mean in decision-making about sexual relationships, thus constructing people with intellectual disabilities as completely incapable of consenting (unless of course they are married). Determining consent, as Gill (2010: 205) notes, is a notoriously difficult exercise, implying engagement with a range of different sets of knowledge including 'legal issues as well as the social, biological and moral meanings and consequences of sexual activities'. Legally, there is divergence across jurisdictions in how consent is understood, or who is to determine it, and whilst scales have been developed to assess capacity to consent, in some cases, overall determinations are made that people with intellectual disabilities do not have capacity to consent at all (Gill 2010). This is currently the case in the Irish context, where capacity legislation dates back to the Lunacy Regulation (Ireland) Act 1871: this Act operates on a status-based notion of capacity, in which someone can be made a Ward of Court, and all decision-making power is taken away from them in every arena of their life: one either has capacity or does not. An outline of a new Mental Capacity Bill, which will introduce a functional-based approach to capacity,[3] was outlined in 2008, but to date the Bill has not yet been enacted. The absence of such legislation is acting as a key stumbling block in Ireland being able to ratify the United Nations' Convention on the Rights of Persons with Disabilities.

Currently, then, in terms of Section 5, people with intellectual disabilities are constructed as legally unable to understand what the sexual act is, or the consequences of such an act; similarly, they are seen as unable to cognitively and emotionally process what sexual desire is or might be. The conspicuous absence of consent within the legislation is as Shildrick (2007a: 55) would suggest 'management by nonrecognition': the silence surrounding it should not be interpreted as benign, nor meaningless, but rather as meaning*ful* insofar as it indicates a discomfort at the notion of people with intellectual disabilities being sexual subjects. Law's overwhelming function to protect fails to recognise sexual identity and expression, and different types of capacities in different circumstances. The challenges presented by this have also become very evident in cases where people with intellectual disabilities have been subjected to sexual abuse and called as witnesses: in many cases, the overwhelming sense of incapacity ascribed to them by the law (or lack of law in this area) has meant that people with intellectual disabilities have been seen as unreliable witnesses and often deemed to be incompetent to give evidence in court (Edwards *et al.* 2012). One might question, then, the effectiveness of pieces of legislation such as Section 5 which work so overwhelmingly off understandings of incapable minds and bodies.

The legal status of sex in place

Whilst law creates particular legal subjectivities and identities and ascribes values to (disabled) body/mind as a site in its own right, so it also contributes to emplacing these bodies, influencing and constructing how the sexuality of people with intellectual disabilities is practised and played out. As geographies of impairment have shown, people's embodied experiences are transformed in and through space: what society may perceive, or react to, as an abnormal or 'out of control' body in one spatial context (for example, in the public sphere) may be experienced as something quite different in another (Moss and Dyck 2002; Parr 2008). As Tyner (2012) also notes, spaces are made, and come into being, through bodily interactions. Thus, the coming together of people in different sites, and at different times, has a potentially transformative effect on the nature of space.

These spatial transmutations become apparent in the way Section 5 of the Criminal Law (Sexual Offences) Act 1993 seeks to locate people with intellectual disabilities in terms of sexual relationships. Historically, legislation regarding sexual offences in most common law countries sought to protect people from rape and other forms of sexual assault in the public arena. However, the way in which these codes of behaviour are applied in the context of the private realm (the home or domestic space, or as Sanger (2001) points out in her aforementioned analysis, the car) has always been subject to greater contestation. Suk (2006: 5) notes how 'the idea that criminal law may not reach into this quintessentially private space has been rightly criticized for enabling the state's acquiescence in violence against women'. Feminist researchers and campaigners have been very successful in bringing domestic violence into the public sphere, and also challenging the assumption that marriage equates with consensual sex. For some, however, this act of bringing into public view the private realm has been almost too successful, such that criminal law has increased its reach into the private sphere of intimate relations, thereby changing spatial practices of the home (Suk 2006).

These debates about the inhabited spaces of intimate human relationships have particular resonance in the case of Section 5. Sexual relationships, and the sexual act itself, is one of the most private and intimate areas of human life: an act which for most people takes place in the private sphere or behind closed doors. The difficulty of constructing intellectually disabled bodies as sexually vulnerable is that it perceives private spaces purely as sites of danger, threat and exploitation for people with intellectual disabilities: more than that, it cannot perceive people with intellectual disabilities in these spaces without law's regulatory reach. In a situation where two people with intellectual disabilities may be cohabiting, for example, the home, or the private realm, is constructed as an unlawful sexual space, a site of risk in which one or both individuals may become offenders. This intrusion into the private sphere that Section 5 engenders is perhaps not surprising given the widespread history of institutionalisation that has existed in Ireland, and the extent to which, even in community settings, the privacy of people with intellectual disabilities is constantly mediated by carers, staff and/or family members (Hollomotz 2009). However, it is one in which the need to protect people with intellectual disabilities overwhelms any notion of supporting their desires for fulfilling sexual expression.

There is, of course, one exception to the legal creation of sexual vulnerability under Section 5, and that is that it allows for a sexual relationship between two people (either between two people with intellectual disabilities, or one person who has an intellectual disability and another who does not) if the two people are married. Marriage therefore acts as a safeguard of some kind of private life, and a proxy for consensual sexual relations in the domestic sphere. In this case, we see two judgments being made. The first of these is a moral value: sex can only take place in and through the institution of marriage, thereby reinforcing traditional moral (and one might add, patriarchal) ideals. The second embodies an assumption that capacity to consent to marriage also means capacity to consent to sex. This in itself is a highly contested issue, and one with which the Law Reform Commission has also concerned itself in seeking to revise Section 5: indeed, in reviewing the legislation, it came to the conclusion that the assessment of whether an individual had the capacity to consent to sexual relations ought to reflect civil law judgments about capacity to marry, and similarly that 'capacity to marry should generally include capacity to consent to sexual relations' (Law Reform Commission 2011: 66). Yet even where an individual does have the capacity to consent to marry and to have sex, it does not mean that rape and sexual assault cannot occur in this domestic private realm.

Section 5, then, whilst making judgments about particular spaces as safe or risky, fails to appreciate the contested notion of space, and not only that, how people may also seek to resist and transform different spaces as the site of intimate sexual relations. The Act seeks to address the 'problem' of people with intellectual disabilities' contested sexuality from a normative standpoint in which sexuality is based on 'a monogamous relation between two adults of opposite genders whose sexual practice is conducted in private and is primarily genitally and reproductively based' (Shildrick 2007a: 56–57). This raises particular issues for those whose sexuality does not conform to such (moral) frameworks, or who inhabit spaces which make 'normal' sexual practices difficult to achieve. For example, there are significant questions for people with intellectual disabilities who continue to live in residential settings regarding how (if at all) they are able to create sites of privacy within such disciplined, segregated arenas. Hollomotz's (2008: 93) research in this area has shown how the failure to provide or respect the private space of people with intellectual disabilities leads them to engage in sexual activity in outside, semi-private spaces, away from public view. Sexual acts then become rushed, and 'individuals have limited time to consider whether they consent to a proposed sexual act and to communicate their decision. Inevitably this places them at risk'. For people with intellectual disabilities in Ireland, moreover, this may involve occupying or creating a legally transgressive and/or criminalised space. Section 5 clearly does not perceive such institutional settings as places where legitimate, or consensual, sexual relationships may form, but neither does it recognise that the lack of privacy may also contribute to risk.[4] The legislation works off what Hollomotz (2009) describes as an individualised notion of vulnerability, without recognising how other socio-cultural, environmental and indeed spatial factors contribute to risk of sexual abuse for people with intellectual disabilities: this in a context where it has been suggested that people with intellectual disabilities are often at higher risk of abuse in residential care settings (McGee *et al.* 2002).

The discussion of Section 5 then demonstrates how disabled bodies/minds become a key site at which the 'law–space nexus' gets worked out in the ordering of sexuality, a nexus which reflects a mutually constitutive relationship between law and space. Law envisions the types of spaces in which people with intellectual disabilities are appropriately able to inhabit as far as their sexuality is concerned, and those which they are not. We see particularly how in the case of Section 5, criminal law encroaches on private spaces and relationships, and indeed, even *eradicates* private space for people with disabilities as far as their sexual relationships are concerned. That said, people with intellectual disabilities may re-author other spaces in order to satisfy their sexual desires, albeit that this involves transgressing legal codes and potentially placing themselves at greater risk. This begs a broader question: *where is* private space for people with intellectual disabilities and how can it be facilitated?

Conclusion

Since the mid 1990s, geographers' engagement with corporeality has sought to bring into view the body/mind as a site intimately bound up with socio-spatial relations: the body/mind affects how we interact with our environment and in turn becomes a site for the inscription of societal values and norms. In this chapter, I have attempted to show how law is one of a set of transformative relations which mediates the identities and spatialities of the impaired body/mind. Legal processes and statutes imprint bodies/minds as spaces in their own right (deeming them capable or incapable, able to consent or not consent in the context of sexual relations, for example), but also affects the way in which they interact with different spaces. Section 5 of the Criminal Law (Sexual Offences) Act 1993 in many ways acts to eradicate private space for people with intellectual disabilities, or sees them solely as vulnerable in private spaces. Meanwhile, the engagement of two people with intellectual disabilities in a sexual act outside marriage creates a transgressive legal space. Marriage is supposed to act as a protective safeguard to the private domain, but as commentators have acknowledged, the Act does not consider what happens within a marriage if one person is no longer able to consent to sexual relations, nor recognises how the private sphere of the home can also be a site of violence (Kelly *et al.* 2009; Suk 2006).

Such legal prescriptions are not 'given', however. As authors such as Parr (2008) have noted, people with disabilities (and indeed other groups) continually seek to resist and re-author perceptions of their bodies/minds and the spaces which they inhabit. People with disabilities are increasingly making calls for their sexuality to be recognised, whilst in Ireland, Section 5 has not stopped service-providing agencies making sex education available to people with intellectual disabilities at a local level, despite fears that an expressed sex education policy might be seen as encouraging law-breaking behaviour. Neither law nor space, then, is a static relation: the law is interpreted in different ways in different places and people interpret and sometimes resist legal definitions and subjectivities in diverse ways. The manner in which the law matters in people's everyday lives, and the ways in which people give meaning to the law – described by some commentators as 'legal consciousness' (Ewick and Silbey 1998; Levine and Mellema 2001) – is an area which arguably requires greater investigation in terms of the sexual lives of people with disabilities.

In the context of this chapter, such investigation is particularly important given the changing spaces within which people with intellectual disabilities are living their lives. Recent policy developments in services for people with intellectual disabilities in Ireland are stressing the move away from living in 'congregated settings' (Health Service Executive 2011), whilst developments in civil law, such as the Disability Act 2005, work from a basis of people with disabilities being 'equal citizens'. These developments are markedly at odds with the emphasis of criminal law in this area. Indeed, Section 5 can be situated within a set of discourses dominated by paternalistic understandings of disability, in which concerns about rights to sexual expression are non-existent: it reflects the thinking of a time in which institutionalised living served as society's answer to the disruption presented by the intellectually impaired body/mind (and did not seek to ask what went on behind these closed doors: private space was seemingly antithetical to living in such settings).

Individuals' claims for their bodies as sites of sexual expression, and policy shifts towards making space for people with intellectual disabilities living in the 'community' may lead to an increased unsettling of conventional societal norms around sexual behaviour and expression. As Shildrick (2007a) notes in the context of debates about independent living and direct payments, for example, calls from disabled people to be facilitated to have sex (either through visiting a sex worker, or facilitated by their personal assistant) feed into debates about the role of the state in supporting disabled people (is it there to support needs *and* desires through welfare payments for example?) as well as broader sexual attitudes. As she states, 'facilitated sex – which by definition cannot be private or self-directed – all too clearly draws attention to the difference of anomalous bodies' (Shildrick 2007a: 60). It is this difference – and the shifting spaces of intimate relations – that law will have to negotiate as it seeks to balance the rights of people with intellectual disabilities to freedom of sexual expression, with their protection from sexual abuse and exploitation.

Notes

1 Throughout the chapter, I refer to the bodies/minds of people with intellectual disabilities, rather than just 'the body'. Much literature on the body, or embodiment, has emerged as a response to the Cartesian dualism which suggested a split between mind and body, in which the former is separate from, and privileged over, the latter. Studies which attempt to 'bring the body back in' are sometimes ambiguous about whether the mind is conceptualised as part of the body. However, I would argue that an awareness of 'the mind' is vital in understanding attitudes towards people with intellectual disabilities' sexuality: perceptions of a 'faulty' mind often lead to an assumption that, as Bacchi and Beasley (2002) note, people do not have autonomous control over their bodies (or that they are controlled by their bodies). I therefore view the mind and body as inherently intertwined and connected, whether we understand them as physical (biological) entities, social entities, or something in between. Whilst I return to conceptualisations of the body/mind later in the chapter, I think Tony Crossley's (2001: 3) definition is a helpful one: 'Human beings are neither minds, nor, strictly speaking, bodies ... but rather mindful and embodied social agents'.

2 I draw heavily in this chapter on feminist literature on the body/mind and sexuality, as a way of interrogating the sexual positioning of *disabled* bodies/minds: insights from feminist geography and also feminist socio-legal scholars open up fruitful lines of inquiry which have marked parallels with 'geographies of disability'. That said, this chapter does not utilise gender as an analytic frame, although I am very conscious of significant work which has brought to the fore the intersection of disability and gender in the experience of violence (see for example, Ortoleva and Lewis' (2012) study of violence against disabled women).

3 A functional approach to capacity implies one in which capacity to make decisions, or understand consequences of decisions, is assessed in the context of specific times and circumstances.

4 Indeed, the legislation has arguably been detrimental in terms of health and social care agencies providing sex education to people with intellectual disabilities in Ireland; as Kelly *et al.* (2009) note, the fear of staff within agencies being seen to encourage people with intellectual disabilities in potentially law-breaking behaviour has had a limiting effect on the extent to which such education is provided (or at least, publicly stated that it is provided).

References

Bacchi, C L and Beasley, C 2002, 'Citizen bodies: is embodied citizenship a contradiction in terms?', *Critical Social Policy*, vol. 22, pp. 324–352.

Berti, M 2010, 'Handcuffed access: homelessness and the justice system', *Urban Geography*, vol. 31, pp. 825–841.

Block, P 2000, 'Sexuality, fertility and danger: twentieth century images of women with cognitive disabilities', *Sexuality and Disability*, vol. 18, pp. 239–254.

Blomley, N K 1989, 'Text and context: rethinking the law-space nexus', *Progress in Human Geography*, vol. 13, pp. 512–534.

Blomley, N K and Bakan, J C 1992, 'Spacing out: towards a critical geography of law', *Osgoode Hall L.J.*, vol. 30, pp. 661–690.

Bordo, S 1993, *Unbearable weight: feminism, western culture and the body*, University of California Press, Berkeley.

Butler, C 2009, 'Critical legal studies and the politics of space', *Social and Legal Studies*, vol. 18, pp. 313–332.

Chouinard, V 1994, 'Geography, law and legal struggles: which ways ahead?', *Progress in Human Geography*, vol. 18, pp. 415–440.

Chouinard, V 1999, 'Life at the margins: disabled women's explorations of ableist spaces', in E K Teather (ed.), *Embodied geographies: spaces, bodies and rites of passage*, Routledge, London, pp. 142–156.

Chouinard, V, Hall, E and Wilton, R 2010, 'Introduction: towards enabling geographies', in V Chouinard, E Hall and R Wilton (eds), *Towards enabling geographies: 'disabled' bodies and minds in society and space*, Ashgate, Aldershot, pp. 1–22.

Cristian, L, Stinson, J and Dotson, L A 2001, 'Staff values regarding the sexual expression of women with developmental disabilities', *Sexuality and Disability*, vol. 19, pp. 283–291.

Crossley, T 2001, *The social body: habit, identity and desire*, Sage, London.

Delaney, D, Ford, R T and Blomley, N 2001, 'Preface: where is law?', in N Blomley, D Delaney and R T Ford (eds), *The legal geographies reader*, Blackwell, Oxford, pp. xiii–xxii.

Dyck, I 2010, 'Geographies of disability: reflections on new body knowledges', in V Chouinard, E Hall and R Wilton (eds), *Towards enabling geographies: 'disabled' bodies and minds in society and space*, Ashgate, Aldershot, pp. 253–263.

Edwards, C and Imrie, R 2003, 'Disability and bodies as bearers of value', *Sociology*, vol. 37, pp. 239–256.

Edwards, C, Harold, G and Kilcommins, S 2012, *Access to justice for people with disabilities as victims of crime in Ireland, Cork*, School of Applied Social Studies/Centre for Criminal Justice and Human Rights, University College, Cork.

Ewick, P and Silbey, S 1998, *The common place of law: stories from everyday life*, University of Chicago Press, Chicago.

Gill, M 2010, 'Rethinking sexual abuse, questions of consent, and intellectual disability', *Sexuality Research and Social Policy*, vol. 7, pp. 201–213.

Government of Ireland 1935, *Criminal Law Amendment Act 1935*, accessed 26 April 2013, www.irishstatutebook.ie/1935/en/act/pub/0006/print.html#sec1.

Government of Ireland 1993, *Criminal Law (Sexual Offences) Act*, accessed 26 April 2013, www.irishstatutebook.ie/1993/en/act/pub/0020/.

Hall, E 2000, '"Blood, brain and bones": taking the body seriously in the geography of health and impairment', *Area*, vol. 32, pp. 21–29.

Health Service Executive 2011, *Time to move on from congregated settings: a strategy for community inclusion report of the working group on congregated settings*, Health Service Executive, Dublin.

Hollomotz, A 2008, '"May we please have sex tonight?" – people with learning difficulties pursuing privacy in residential group settings', *British Journal of Learning Disabilities*, vol. 37, pp. 91–97.

Hollomotz, A 2009, 'Beyond "vulnerability": an ecological model approach to conceptualizing risk of sexual violence against people with learning difficulties', *British Journal of Social Work*, vol. 39, pp. 99–112.

Hughes, B and Paterson, K 1997, 'The social model of disability and the disappearing body: towards a sociology of impairment', *Disability and Society*, vol. 12, pp. 325–340.

Imrie, R and Edwards, C 2007, 'Geographies of disability: reflections on the development of a sub-discipline', *Geography Compass*, vol. 1, pp. 623–640.

Johnston, L and Longhurst, R 2010, *Space, place and sex: geographies of sexualities*, Rowman & Littlefield, Lanham.

Kelly, G, Crowley, H and Hamilton, C 2009, 'Rights, sexuality and relationships in Ireland: "It'd be nice to be kind of trusted"', *British Journal of Learning Disabilities*, vol. 37, pp. 308–315.

Law Reform Commission 1990, *Report on sexual offences against the mentally handicapped*, LRC 33–1990, Law Reform Commission, Dublin.

Law Reform Commission 2011, *Sexual offences and capacity to consent: consultation paper*, LRC CP 63 – 2011, Law Reform Commission, Dublin.

Levine, K and Mellema, V 2001, 'Strategizing the street: how law matters in the lives of women in the street-level drug economy', *Law and Social Inquiry*, vol. 26, pp. 169–207.

Longhurst, R 1997, '(Dis)embodied geographies', *Progress in Human Geography*, vol. 21, pp. 486–501.

Longhurst, R 1999, 'Pregnant bodies, public scrutiny: "giving" advice to pregnant women', in E K Teather (ed.), *Embodied geographies: spaces, bodies and rites of passage*, Routledge, London, pp. 77–90.

Longhurst, R 2001, 'Geography and gender: looking back, looking forward', *Progress in Human Geography*, vol. 25, pp. 641–648.

Longhurst, R 2010, 'The disabling affects of fat: the emotional and material geographies of some women who live in Hamilton, New Zealand', in V Chouinard, E Hall and R Wilton (eds), *Towards enabling geographies: 'disabled' bodies and minds in society and space*, Ashgate, Aldershot, pp. 199–216.

Lupton, D 2012, 'Configuring maternal, preborn and infant embodiment', *Sydney Health and Society Group Working Paper No.2*, Sydney Health and Society Group, Sydney.

McCarthy, M and Thompson, D 1996, 'Sexual abuse by design: an examination of issues in learning disability services', *Disability and Society*, vol. 11, pp. 205–218.

McDonnell, P 2007, *Disability and society: ideological and historical dimensions*, Blackhall Publishing, Dublin.

McGee, H, Garavna, R, de Barra, M, Byrne, J and Conroy, R 2002, *The SAVI report: sexual abuse and violence in Ireland*, Liffey Press, Dublin.

Mitchell, D 2001, 'The annihilation of space by law: the roots and implications of anti-homeless laws in the United States', in N Blomley, D Delaney and R T Ford (eds), *The legal geographies reader*, Blackwell, Oxford, pp. 6–18.

Morin, K M and Berg, L D 1999, 'Emplacing current trends in feminist historical geography', *Gender, Place and Culture*, vol. 6, pp. 311–330.

Moss, P and Dyck, I 2002, *Women, body, illness: space and identity in the everyday lives of women with chronic illness*, Rowman & Littlefield, Lanham.

National Disability Authority 2011, *A national survey of public attitudes to disability in Ireland*, NDA, Dublin.

Ortoleva, S and Lewis, H 2012, 'Forgotten sisters: a report on violence against women with disabilities: an overview of its nature, scope, causes and consequences', *Northeastern*

Public Law and Theory Faculty Research Paper Series No. 104–2012, Northeastern University, Boston.

Parr, H 2008, *Mental health and social space: towards inclusionary geographies*, Blackwell, Oxford.

Rich, A 1986, *Blood, bread and poetry: selected prose 1979–1985*, Norton, New York.

Sanger, C 2001, 'Girls and the getaway: cars, culture and the predicament of gendered space', in N Blomley, D Delaney and R T Ford (eds), *The legal geographies reader*, Blackwell, Oxford, pp. 31–41.

Shildrick, M 2007a, 'Contested pleasures: the socio-political economy of disability and sexuality', *Sexuality Research and Social Policy: Journal of NSRC*, vol. 4, pp. 53–66.

Shildrick, M 2007b, 'Dangerous discourses: anxiety, desire and disability', *Studies in Gender and Sexuality*, vol. 8, pp. 221–244.

Smart, C 1989, *Feminism and the power of law*, Routledge, London.

Sobsey, M 1994, *Violence and abuse in the lives of people with disabilities: the end of silent acceptance?*, Paul H. Brookes, Baltimore.

Suk, J 2006, 'Criminal law comes home', *The Yale Law Journal*, vol. 116, no. 1, pp. 2–70.

Teather, E K 1999, 'Introduction: geographies of personal discovery', in E K Teather (ed.), *Embodied geographies: spaces, bodies and rites of passage*, Routledge, London, pp. 1–26.

Tremain, S 2005, 'Foucault, governmentality and critical disability theory', in S Tremain (ed.), *Foucault and the government of disability*, University of Michigan Press, Michigan, pp. 1–24.

Tyner, J A 2012, *Space, place and violence: violence and the embodied geographies of race, sex and gender*, Routledge, London.

Walmsley, J 2000, 'Women and the Mental Deficiency Act of 1913: citizenship, sexuality and regulation', *British Journal of Learning Disabilities*, vol. 28, pp. 65–70.

3   The spaces of poverty

Renegotiating place and disability in the global South

Shaun Grech

Introduction

The subject of disability in the global South has gained some currency in recent years framed as a new field called 'disability and development' or 'global disability'. Much of these developments have happened within disciplines such as global health and anthropology, and engagement with disability has come through attempts at creating linkages between disability and international development, an area with a stated global South focus (see for example Maclachlan and Swartz 2009). Arguments have emerged suggesting that disability cuts across all of the Millennium Development Goals (MDGs) and, hence, cannot be excluded from the global development agenda (Mulligan and Gooding 2009). The move towards a rights-based approach to development was another point of connection (see Stubbs 2008). It has been, though, the frequently alluded to relationship between disability and poverty that has provided the strongest linkages between disability and development (see WHO and World Bank 2011).[1]

But while there has been a growing body of literature on disability in the global South since the mid 1990s (in particular in global health), disability continues to be excluded from development policy, practice and research.[2] The current attempts at including disability in the Post-2015 MDG Framework are a clear testimony of this. There remains a dearth of empirical material looking at the dynamics operating between disability and poverty (Grech 2009), and a substantial amount of the literature around disability in the global South remains grey literature (in particular documents and reports by international organisations). Much of this literature echoes discourses and 'findings' from other areas or pertinent to high visibility populations within the development sector, such as women, people with HIV/AIDS, and racial and ethnic minorities. Disability is often cast into the faceless category 'vulnerable' within the development sector, an ontological all-encompassing space, a kind of limbo for all those who do not 'fit' among the productive poor, not here or there, but are seen as being in need of some other 'intervention'. While disabled people are seldom mentioned, the notions of vulnerability and the deserving poor continue to create the impression that disabled people are somehow included in the development space. Over the years, this category has, and continues to, legitimise a cadre of experts and organisations, determining funding priorities and programmes. As Satterthwaite (2008: xii) emphasises:

> professionals of all kinds need vulnerable groups, just as the police need criminals ... to characterise a group as vulnerable is to lay claim to a specialism ... and to construct the individual or group as vulnerable in the sense of having a peculiar need which only this expertise can meet.

If we were to take seriously the guesstimate that around 80 per cent of disabled people are located in the global South (WHO and World Bank 2011), then one would believe that disability studies would have long prioritised the lives of disabled people within the global South. Unfortunately, though, the field remains the arena of global North (read British and US) academics, with solid white, Western, middle-class foundations retaining an almost exclusive focus on the global North. The global South (real or imagined) remains confined to a space of distance, perhaps even irrelevance, within this Northern-dominated field. In spite of this, a pattern that has emerged in recent years has been one of exportation (sometimes imposition) of Western disability tenets, epistemologies and discourse, with little or no alertness to these contexts imbued with spatial and temporal complexities and heterogeneities.[3] While much of this exportation happens at the hands of international and national organisations (endorsing the 'latest' enlightened Western discourse), many disability studies scholars and activists encourage this process even in subtle ways. This dynamic has triggered some critique in recent years, including the charge of epistemic neocolonisation (see Grech 2009, 2011; Meekosha 2011).

But this is not the only problem in the global disability landscape. A worrying pattern that remains is the lack of interdisciplinary interaction between fields such as disability studies, global health, anthropology and international development. On the one hand global health sustains its efforts at epidemiological and other work and at putting disability on the development map, it continues to shy away from theoretical and critical work such as that in critical disability studies. On the other hand, international development struggles to create connections between its work on poverty and the relevance of disability to this work, and to start engaging with other disciplines that do. While some have started to speak about 'global disability', the general lack of interdisciplinary dialogue (among other reasons), means that there is no such thing as a 'global disability studies' yet.

In this chapter I respond to, and critically challenge, some of these emerging concerns as Western disability studies confront the Southern space, in particular the transfer of discourse and practice from global North to global South. To articulate and highlight these concerns, I will be drawing from ongoing ethnographic research in Guatemala. This chapter does not intend (nor is it possible) to provide an exhaustive critique. Instead, it is one small effort at creating a dialogue on critical issues cross-cutting different fields.

On the power of place: the complex majority world and the power of Western 'knowledge'

Before engaging with some of the critical emerging issues, it is, though, best to start off with how the majority world or the global South is approached (if at all) by Western disability theorists. Reading mainstream texts (see for example Barnes and Mercer 2002; Davis 2010; Oliver 1996), one is immediately struck by two patterns. The first pattern is the virtual absence of the global South from any of the content. Not only are the lives of disabled people within these spaces ignored, but there is an almost complete disengagement from Southern epistemologies and work by Southern disability theorists. These Western writings, largely pitched as the leading disability studies texts (worked out in enlightened Western institutions to be disseminated to others round the globe), consistently disregard any disability literature in these dark, distant places, in particular those not writing in the dominant English language, the *lingua franca* (e.g. Latin American theorists). Many are also using literature, discourse and even writing styles that are different, not considered acceptable alongside the rest of the chapters (e.g. in an edited text such as this one) or the dominant disability studies discourse. The exclusion of these not only retains the exclusivity and dominance of Western disability studies writings, but it subjugates Southern knowledge, the Southern space and voice, sustaining a disability studies, often insular, sometimes limited in its scope and breadth.

But the general approach of shifting ideas from the West to the rest is not new (see Santos 2012). Instead, it reflects the continued dominance of Western knowledge, practices and institutions, the unfettered control over what counts as knowledge, and how it is produced, by whom, and how it should be disseminated. This power is not limited to creating an academic idiom, but is a function of, and propagates, broader power asymmetries accrued over history, maintaining a periphery eternally subjugated to the knowledge of the Northern. It is these asymmetries that ultimately permit the globalisation of knowledge, which as Habashi (2005) argues, is invariably from North to South. This failure to account for epistemological diversity, and 'the location of the Southern disabled body within North-South power relations' (Soldatic and Biyanwila 2010: 77) leaves the disability knowledge system unchallenged, unchanged and, more than anything, limits theoretical developments in Eurocentric disability studies imaginings. As Santos (2012: 45) notes, though, this condition is not unique to disability studies alone:

> social theories produced in the global North are not necessarily universally valid, even when they purport to be general theories … the theories produced in the global North are best equipped to account for the social, political and cultural realities of the global North and … in order to account for the realities of the global South other theories must be developed and anchored in other epistemologies – the epistemologies of the South.

The second pattern is the token inclusion of the majority world as a last or isolated chapter (see for example the *Handbook of disability studies* by Albrecht *et al.*

2001), a global South fixed at the ontological fringes. In spite of this, the word 'global' is quickly becoming an opportunistic stint to enhance the attraction of disability studies texts to publishers, and to sell the idea that the perspectives inside are relevant to all (global reach = more sizable market). Furthermore, 'those' parts of the world pitched as 'lacking' (including in literature) are also accommodated (via an 'inclusive' text), implying that they, too, can become potential customers. Still, and contemporaneously, it leaves the North to South globalisation of knowledge unchanged, and in practice, few of these texts include global South writers.[4]

There are commonalities between these two patterns. The first is an inordinate homogenising of the global South space and its people, neatly packaged by Western theorists (flirting with global disability issues) as an almost undifferentiated space, because this makes it discursively manageable and controllable (see Said 1979). This is especially the case when this space has hardly been contemplated, and when the theories deployed (e.g. the social model) have not been written with the majority world in mind (or issues therein), but which are nevertheless made to 'fit' every corner of the world. This embodies the familiar dynamic of 'benevolent but imperialist universalism' (Santos 2012: 46). Indeed, the complexities and heterogeneities (socio-economic, political, historical, cultural, ideological, religious/spiritual) that make up the hybrid global South (including within countries) are too often ignored, removed or resisted. I discuss some of these aspects below. Within this pattern, one also finds a frequent homogenisation of the disability experience. Indeed, space and temporality are often streamlined in the bid to create a 'consistent' discourse. In recent years, inferences from the global North about the presumed situation of *all* disabled people in these 'developing' countries have emerged, suggesting that disabled people are inordinately oppressed, ill-treated and almost invariably victims of much suffering in the Southern space. The following example is illustrative: 'Ignorance, fear of impairment and negative attitudes about disabled people mean that they are marginalised and excluded from opportunities for human development' (Barron and Ncube 2010: 2). Flowing through such discourse is the call for outside intervention (knowing/developed/benevolent/civilised) in these spaces and lives (faceless/ignorant/uncivilised, etc.), because 'the native is declared insensible to ethics; he represents not only the absence of values, but also the negation of values' (Fanon 1963: 32).

Streamlining the disability experience through dominant frames, such as the social model of disability or human rights discourse, strengthens the disability metanarrative that feeds back into the legitimacy and perceived relevance of these Northern frames round the four corners of the globe. We see for example a Community Based Rehabilitation (CBR) shipped off as guidelines by global North international organisations, globalising a physical and mental health regime mapped out by the World Health Organisation (WHO). But there is still little questioning as to the possible role of CBR in sustaining a neoliberal development sector thirsty for strong productive bodies, which, above all, are not a costly burden. One is also hard-pressed to question the extent to which 'community' and notions of social capital are little more than opportunistic 'rediscoveries' in a development sector bent on cost-cutting, privatisation, and where the idea of community means little more than autonomous people taking care of themselves, unburdening governments (see Grech 2010).[5]

Most critically, the geopolitical asymmetries permitting the movement/imposition of epistemologies and practice from global North to global South are rarely, if ever, questioned. This maintains not only an epistemological void around such issues, but also the sense of legitimacy/obligation to continue 'educating', 'giving' or rather transferring. The 'global' sells, but the historical baggage (in particular the colonial) that endows the neoliberal globalisation of knowledge and practices, replete with inequality and epistemic violence, is hardly interrogated in disability studies, (re-)inscribing the post/neocolonising of the Southern space, subject and knowledge.

It is easy to see the paradox, where out of convenience, commonalities are easily sought between global North and South (and within the South) if these permit the shipping off of global North epistemologies and practices. But when it comes to asserting superiority, whether of the Western disability studies discourse, or the global North institutions teaching them, differences are quickly outlined and the South constructed as Other. This is the moment where 'the misery of the Third World is the result of its own incompetence, its own inanity – in short, of its *subhumanity*' (Badiou 2002: 13, italics in original). This process is sustained by a dynamic of erasure of what there was, is and could ever be in these distant dark spaces across time, a dynamic that not only sustains the domination of these Western values and their institutions, it also removes the possibility that the South could ever have anything of value to contribute to the metanarratives of the superior Northern space.[6] And again the imperialistic trail of Western 'knowledge' and practices, the academic neocolonalism continues unabated, an 'epistemic violence' predicated on the positioning of the native 'perceived outside the normative subject of Western modernity' (Cutajar 2008: 29). Approaches of 'essentialism and exclusiveness, or with barriers and sides' such as these, as Said stressed, 'give rise to polarizations that absolve and forgive ignorance and demagogy more than they enable knowledge' (1993: 35).

In the 'spaces of poverty' is a disability that is lived in complex places

The dynamics highlighted above give rise to a plethora of issues, which are impossible to address in this chapter. Instead, I will be engaging with some critical concerns emerging from the lack or absence of engagement with the Southern space (material and discursive) by Western disability studies. Critically, I am interested in how this space, in its full fluidity, complexity and heterogeneity, not only interacts with, but importantly (re-)constructs, disability in ways that profoundly challenge Western epistemologies and, more basically, 'knowledge', redefining a Southern space imbued with agency and resistance to the 'Eurocentric paradigm' of 'truth', 'order' and 'reality' (Pisani 2013). Engaging with the Southern space is not a luxury for any credible analysis or theory because disabled people and their families live and are constructed within/through it.

Engaging with the Southern space means engaging with poverty, which, despite its own complexities and multi-dimensionalities, is often a critical presence within this space. Unfortunately, though, it is also this poverty that is assumed, simplified and often generalised from North to South within the Western disability studies (see for example Barnes and Sheldon 2010). Indeed, the word 'poverty' is quickly adopted, attempting to create the impression that we all know what is being talked about, or that indeed, it is all the same type of poverty, and hence there is no need to define or problematise it. But this is a profound contradiction when it is this same assumed (and disproportionate perhaps different) poverty that (to many) defines the 'global South' as a space constructed as ontologically separate or Other to what they know as the West or global North (itself often simplified, homogenised and dehistoricised).[7] Furthermore the call for 'poverty eradication' in development perpetually (re-)constructs the Southern space as one that is needing, and perhaps even desiring, intervention (see Botello 2005).[8]

This poverty, though, is stripped of historicity, in particular the geopolitical asymmetries that created, sustain and perpetuate it. Indeed, as disability studies is confronted with the Southern space, few are the attempts at considering the colonial encounter and its implications for a disability, which, like poverty, is constructed and lived historically, consistently traversing the past as it navigates into the future (Grech 2011). While colonialism lies deep in the psyche of both coloniser and colonised, there are not only different propensities (if at all) to recollect it, but critically, different memories and interpretations of the 'civilising' mission.

But even more practically, what poverty means in very specific places is seldom engaged with. Indeed, the nuances and complexities of livelihoods, geography and rurality, infrastructure, health systems, social protection, psychological and spiritual dimensions (to name but a few aspects) are hardly considered in the analysis. In empirical work on disability and poverty, even outside disability studies (see for example Barron and Ncube 2010), we are also very rarely provided with any insight into the contexts of poverty and poor people's (including disabled people's) own understandings and interpretations of poverty, and how this is lived and survived. In fact, disability is all too often framed in isolation. This not only contributes to the lack of understanding around the nuances of poverty on the ground, but also feeds back into homogenising the Southern space and legitimising indefinitely dominant epistemologies and practices with little or no consultation with the poor, including disabled people. Examples are many, including the trust placed in disability quotas in contexts where schools are inaccessible to most poor children, and are physically unequipped to deal with the demands of disabled children (e.g. overcrowdedness; lack of teaching materials such as books in Braille). Other examples, and perhaps most obviously, are capacity building and job skills training for disabled people in isolation, without considering the limitations imposed by poverty, including limited disposable income.

Disability needs to be positioned within very specific *spaces of poverty*, spaces that are as material as they are discursive and ontological. These dynamic spaces are critical in understanding how disability is constructed and lived across space and time, but always constitutive of and constituted within/through the poverty space. Spaces of poverty, like the global South, are hybrid, pushing us to problematise boundaries and totalising forms of cultural understandings, knowledge and notions of identity and place at the most basic levels (see Nederveen Pieterse 2001). The Southern space is one where people have for centuries been blending the traditional and the modern, many operating at various and interacting margins (even of globalisation and markets) (see García Canclini 2005). This, though, does not mean that there are no patterns that may look unfamiliar to the Northern outsider fixed within a specific schema. Indeed, positioning disability within these spaces of poverty implies a conscious effort at seeking out and prioritising what may be different from, or even contradict, the homogenising gaze of the Northern disability theorist.

One may include here a number of examples. The majority of people in the global South, and in particular those in extreme poverty (75 per cent), reside in rural areas (IFAD 2011). This often means physical isolation from main thoroughfares, including services such as schools and health care facilities; poor housing and sanitation; vulnerability to natural hazards such as floods and droughts. While the majority (some 80 per cent) depend on agriculture, many of the rural poor are involved in complex and diverse livelihood activities (e.g. collection of water and firewood), which are not always remunerated (e.g. work in kind or sharecropping). Many of these rural poor are often producers and consumers (of their own subsistence crop) contemporaneously. Having one foot in the market and the other in subsistence means (to an extent) that they enter and exit the market but still manage to survive. Most of the labouring activities in these places are performed in the informal sector, implying that the poor are not entitled to regularised work rights (e.g. sick leave and insurance), or social protection (e.g. disability benefits or pensions). The major cost for these poor families is the food basket (around 50 and 70 per cent of the household budget versus 10–15 per cent in rich countries) (FAO 2008), leaving little or no disposable income (including for health care), while price hikes of staples consistently impact food consumption. Poor rural families are not always unitary or blood-related, and do not always share access and control over resources. These rural areas exist within a complex Southern space hosting 1 billion of the world's hungry; where 1.5 million people die every year from diarrhoeal diseases (including cholera); and some 75 million children are out of school (UNESCO 2010; WHO 2009, 2010). The Southern space is also one where religion continues to grow incrementally, for example Christianity (including Evangelical denominations) in Latin America. In fact, the Southern space is far from alien to religion, not least on account of the Christianising missions sustaining and legitimising the brutal colonial enterprise.[9]

Disability in the spaces of poverty: fluid definitions

When disability is placed within these fluid spaces, the idea that 'there is no generally accepted definition of disability' (Pfeiffer 2007: 103), becomes more than credible, and that no single model can encapsulate the disability experience. The meanings of disability, it is clear, are dependent on what is valued in these same spaces (material and ontological), necessitating an understanding of what is conceptualised as full personhood in specific contexts and temporalities, or rather 'the cosmology and values and purposes of life' because 'the cultural conceptualization of humanity is variable' (Whyte and Ingstad 1995: 10, 11). Rather than attempting to frame disability in isolation, one must therefore start by understanding what *surrounds* disability, because this is what disability is positioned along/against and how it is interpreted by both disabled people and those around them.

Notions of personhood are complex since these vary across multiple geographical (e.g. rural and urban), spatial, social, cultural, gender, racial/ethnic and economic dimensions, imbued within broader notions of ideology and spirituality. In rural Guatemala, for men, full personhood often means being married, owning a house, having children, and critically, labouring as the main and often sole breadwinner to support one's family and ensuring survival. The latter forms a critical component in the maintenance of a hegemonic masculinity (Bird 1996). For women, full personhood is about marriage (ideally to a suitable candidate who can support financially), bearing and raising healthy children, attending to household and other tasks, supplementing (not replacing) the husband's labour and earnings, and maintaining familial and social relationships. Cross-cutting these is the importance attributed to family, the most important institution for the poor (see also Narayan *et al.* 2000). Within this, children are socially and culturally valued and expected, since they satisfy emotional needs, enable the continuation of the family, and most critically are the only insurance mechanism possessed by the poor. Within contexts such as these, it is not surprising that disability can mean a range of things, from the inability to provide for one's family, childlessness, to limited resources to provide care for others. The following quote captures some of these aspects:

> Family, and then the children, you give them food, they grow up, so that they can then help you, because there is no government or anything, so like me, my children are not here, I can barely eat, and I cannot feed my wife, so this, my disability, is lived on her body too, because before this, I provided.
>
> (Felipe)

Notions of full personhood need to be firmly positioned within the Southern space and the spaces of poverty. Globally, fate and religion have for centuries provided a plethora of frames around the human condition, in particular meaning-making, influencing perceptions and worldviews (Alkire 2006). A range of authors (see Berghs 2012; Ghai 2002) highlight how religious beliefs are often critical in constructing understandings around impairment and disability, and how they should be lived and 'intervened' in, by both disabled people and those around them, within broader complex spiritual interpretations of embodiment, relationships and nature. The dominance of spiritual-religious readings are perhaps not surprising in contexts where health care is often fragmented or absent, and where medical labels are sparse. In the absence of these, religious beliefs provide meaning-making (including around the provenance of impairment), influence behaviour, and are on occasion also a source of resistance (psychological and material). The following vignettes are illustrative:

> Disability is the will of God, he helps me understand why I am like this, and where I will go.
>
> (Fausto)

> There is only my small church here, nothing else, the congregation helps me emotionally and with some money when I cannot eat … they are the line between this life and the next, because our religion says we should help the weak.
>
> (Maria)

Maria and Fausto's words highlight the importance of beliefs but also challenge at the very core secular disciplines such as the Western disability studies. The need to engage with religion and spirituality are critical since these constitute a key ontological frame traversing the discursive, the cosmological and the material. Indeed, 'freedom of religion is only possible in a world free of religion' (Santos 2009: 4).

Where health care access is absent, it is also no surprise that the embodied experience of disability, in particular pain and impairment, may not only be prioritised, but equated with disability, framed within a discourse needing and even desiring medicalisation. When survival is predicated on harsh physical labour, attention may indeed be refocused on achieving previous body functioning, or the attempt to 'erase any signs of change to … return the body … to a past era of supposed perfection' (Siebers 2010: 328). This highlights first of all the danger of denying the narratives of impairment emanating from bodies which are profoundly social, especially when these narratives struggle to be heard within dominant disability discourses and practices. Livingston (2006: 113), for example, emphasises how 'the marginalization of the somatic aspects of impairment in the field of disability studies contrasted with their emphasis in Botswana'. It also perhaps warrants against indiscriminate attacks on the medicalisation of disability, especially when such discourse may alienate or distance much needed medical care, medication and medical professionals. This is a very serious concern when neoliberal cost-cutting and privatisation continue to mean reduced access to health care and rehabilitation, especially for the poorest people. In such contexts, if anything, health care needs to be not only prioritised, but also theorised and politicised. The following quote articulates not only the focus on pain and the body, but a call for health care capable of diagnosing and 'reducing' some of this pain in order to survive:

> Pain, my body can't survive like this, the first thing I feel and know about myself is that I am damaged, and that my body needs to be fixed … But I first

need to know what is wrong, and then to have a doctor cure me, so that I can work, love, provide for my family and be with others.

(Juan Carlos)

Families and communities of poverty: beyond individual spaces, beyond individual rights

What cuts across much of what is articulated above, is the strong presence and ontological significance of the collective. The spaces of poverty are ones where families and communities remain the most important and valuable institutions, providing access to assets and resources, and often ensuring survival (see Narayan *et al.* 2000). These are contexts where the idea of community exists firmly within people's psyche and lifeworlds, real and imagined, or as Mkhize (2004: 49) suggests, where a person is 'a person-in-relation, a "being-with-and-for-others" and not an isolated atomistic individual'. These are spaces where the private and the public are not dichotomised or so clear-cut.

When much of identity, meaning, representation, resilience and survival are constructed and lived in and through community, we are pushed to question the applicability of the discourse on rights (including disability rights), premised upon the Western fetishising of independence and autonomy. These are spaces where relationships and reciprocity dominate over the immediate demands of the individual, and where it would hence be more adequate to speak about *communal rights* (see also Miles 2000).[10] Within any universalising discourse such as that on human rights are also homogenised notions of: well-being; 'good life'; justice and injustice; dignity; cultural, social and economic dis/integration; racist and discriminating discourse and practice. Above all, standardised recommendations are framed as 'good practice' across the board. But, as Santos questions, 'if humanity is one alone, why are there so many different principles concerning human dignity and a just society, all of them presumably unique, yet often contradictory among themselves?' (2009: 3). Indeed, while policies and conventions (e.g. the UN Convention on the Rights of Persons with Disabilities) are enthusiastically transposed from North to South, not only is there an inherent homogenising of space, but also an opportunistic notion of the world as *one* place (see above). But, and contemporaneously, there is an inherent and arrogant assumption that within the Southern space people do not have their own concepts of social justice regulating their interactions, and most critically have nothing to contribute to the rights discourse on what it means to be a full and 'civilised' human being. There is also an almost complete inattention to communities (e.g. in remote rural areas) living outside this discourse, unknowing of these same policies and their own 'rights' on paper, and who can, much less, on account of their poverty, ever claim their rights and seek redress (Grech 2009). Long-standing cultural beliefs and ideologies are also hard to erase, and people's perceptions, attitudes and behaviours, one can perhaps reflect, will hardly be changed through legislation alone. Instead, they will forever influence the applicability, relevance and limitations of any discourse and practice.

Probing further these communities of poverty, international literature also suggests a plethora of beliefs, responses and attitudes towards disabled people in these hugely complex and varied contexts, including positive ones (see Ingstad and Whyte 2007). Oscar, an indigenous rural participant, highlights aspects of a life shared as a collective, and where survival hinges on the love and care of family and community:

> We eat, we work, we survive together … we cannot pull throughout without our families and communities, they are our brick and mortar … where you have nothing, you have God to warm your soul, and your neighbours to feed your body.
>
> (Oscar)

Where the communal envelopes the individual, we also need to look at the impacts of disability on the whole family, since, in the absence of any formal safety nets, disability is a family responsibility. These impacts are so strong that perhaps we should be speaking about a *disabled family*, necessitating a household analysis, and suggesting that any intervention needs to support all family members, as opposed to the disabled individual in isolation. The following quote highlights a trail of impoverishment and ill-health for family members:

> I needed an operation, so we borrowed the money, at 15% interest, we have nothing, look, so my children had to leave school and go work the fields, my wife is now ill, she had to stop her medication because we couldn't handle the costs of her medicine, repayments for the loan, and food to live … we are poorer and we all need help.
>
> (Mario)

Examples such as this challenge the frequent generalisations in disability discourse around the condition of all disabled people in the global South (see above). While ill-treatment does exist (and there should be local active movements for change), the problem is that such discourse is predicated on the notion of the Southern space and subject as inferior, brutal, in need and even desiring of external intervention. On the contrary, and while oppression and even violence against disabled people happen regularly in the global North, no Northern or even Southern writer would ever contemplate a statement such as 'Disabled People in the West are neglected and killed'. When transposed to the global South, this discourse of ill-treatment and cruelty is indeed *expected*. As Quijano (2008: 190) observes, this approach has strong colonial lineages predicated on racial difference, a perspective of 'imagined modernity and rationality as exclusively European products and experiences'. Instead, the agency, love and care of families are often rendered invisible, while perpetually reconstructing these spaces as ones needing/desiring 'external', 'learned', 'human' intervention. In the short quote below, Katarina reflects on her family, positioned within a rural space of care:

No family is perfect, neither is mine, but they have struggled day after day to keep me alive, with a tortilla, trying to gather some money for a pill for my pain, or to keep some faith in my heart when I am sad … we, unlike those in cities, live together, farm and survive together, we are only humans sharing this space.

(Katarina)

Disability is heterogeneous: (re-)negotiating disability in the dynamic spaces of poverty

Drawing together the sections above, one is left with a scenario of substantial complexity and heterogeneity of the Southern space, subject and disability. Disability and the disability experience are fluid, hybrid and constantly (re-)negotiated across space and time, suggesting a deep suspicion of all-encompassing models or narratives. Disabled people themselves are not a homogeneous group, and their experiences are invariably shaped by other social microcosms, including the type of impairment, gender, religion, age, ethnic/racial group, caste, availability of family support, location, availability of services in proximity, types of livelihoods, ideological, spiritual and religious beliefs, availability (or otherwise) of formal support, and much more (Grech 2009). This feeds back into the notion that rather than singling out disabled people and their condition, any analysis needs to start off with an in-depth understanding of these diverse spaces of poverty and personhood, how disability is constructed and lived in relation/through these spaces, and in turn feeds into (re-)constructing these spaces and even ideas around what it means to be 'non-disabled'. As Weiss (2007: 121) states, 'by questioning the construction of normalcy and problematizing it within specific sociocultural contexts … the issue of abnormality and disability is also questioned and problematized'. For example, subsistence family-based agriculture often provides a wide range of tasks such as seeding and fertilising that accommodate all or most of the poor, including disabled people. In such contexts, a person with dyslexia may not necessarily be disadvantaged in labouring or oppressed. This is opposed to urban areas. But in contexts such as these, where there is little or no access to health care, many face harsher living conditions on account of costs, unmedicated pain, and limited ability to labour (itself necessitating physical strength). This is especially the case for persons with chronic impairments requiring large and consistent amounts of health care. Overall, these impact how disability and poverty are lived by oneself as well as one's family. The following quote articulates the importance of engaging with the diverse spaces of poverty:

You need to understand how we work together the family land, how we share the bean, how I, even with my body like this … try and do some work when not in much pain … but only a bit because if I get hurt I have to buy some medicine, and we cannot afford it, so only a few hours … but at least, here we don't have to pay rent or electricity, so we just try and grow what we eat.

(José)

Conclusion

The message of this chapter is perhaps simple, and more than anything warrants against the tendency to simplify and generalise the global South space, subject and disability experience, especially when our own epistemologies and practices are premised on and developed in specific spaces imbued with a historical baggage of geopolitical asymmetries. Engaging with the spaces of poverty within the complex Southern space necessitates openness and, more than anything, the decolonisation of the debate and discipline to make the global South a key focus and priority.

We urgently need a disability studies that is consistently engaging and learning about these contexts and spaces, a disability studies that is interdisciplinary, (self-) reflexive and open to alternative epistemologies, realities, and ways of knowing, learning and talking about worlds. Within this position, the Southern voices must be consistently heard and prioritised, especially those challenging the fixities of our own positions and practices, since 'if the epistemological diversity of the world is to be accounted for, other theories must be developed and anchored in other epistemologies – the epistemologies of the South that adequately account for the realities of the global South' (Santos 2012: 43).

Capturing the disability experience and defining it through any one meta-narrative is ultimately impossible because contexts and circumstances, including the spaces of poverty, are not static. Indeed, even within single countries, spaces of poverty vary and are dynamic over time, including: level and type of geographical isolation; food availability and levels of hunger; environmental pressures and disasters (e.g. drought impacting agricultural output); conflict; and migration (impacts household labour availability and support, especially for weaker members). The circumstances faced by disabled people and their households are also changing, including: levels and qualities of health care (and hence costs) required; number of dependents (in particular children who themselves need to be educated and fed); and numbers of working children and relatives contributing to household welfare. If the spaces of poverty and the lives therein are fluid and dynamic, this suggests that any analysis of disability within these spaces needs to also be open to change over time, since it is not only the meaning of poverty that is fluid, but also what is conceptualised as full personhood across time, feeding into the notion of *disability as a dynamic human condition*.

Notes

1 For example rough estimates have emerged suggesting that 20 per cent of the world's poorest are disabled people (WHO and World Bank 2011).
2 Indeed, a review of mainstream development journals and textbooks reveals content that is practically free of disability.
3 In the international arena, the most visible of these have perhaps been the social model of disability, individual rights and independent living.
4 Instead, these are often limited to chapters by people such as myself (based in a global North university writing in English) to add a 'global' flavour to texts that ultimately remain profoundly global North oriented and fixed.

5 To be clear, tools such as the social model have and continue to do much to politicise disability and sustain the efforts of activists worldwide – and are far from irrelevant. What I am arguing about here is the need to engage with what is forsaken when epistemologies and practices are exported indiscriminately with little or no alertness or sensitivity to other spatial and contextual locations. Above all, it is the fact that these are rarely exported on people's own terms – we are indeed still to see the emergence of an African or Latin American social model of disability or disability studies altogether.

6 Santos (2009: 104) notes how the: '"West" ... managed to impose its conceptions of past and future, of time and space, on the rest of the world. It has thus made its values and institutions prevail, turning them into expressions of western exceptionalism, thereby concealing similarities and continuities with values and institutions existing in other regions of the world'. He goes on to state that the best way to combat Eurocentrism is 'to show that all the things attributed to the West as being exceptional and unique ... have parallels and antecedents in other world regions and cultures' noting further how 'the West's preponderance, therefore, cannot be explained by means of categorical differences, but rather by means of processes of elaboration and intensification' (104).

7 To emphasise, I am not dichotomising global North and global South. Indeed there are/ have been multiple fusions and dynamic movements of ideas as well as material practices in all directions. What I am speaking about are some of the dimensions constituting the ontological construction of the global South, of which poverty is one critical dimension, sometimes also in Othering this space. Despite the fusions and similarities, economic and other inequalities do exist, are often skewed in favour of the metropole, highlighting not only an unequal playing field, but also the political, social, historical, cultural and ideological factors and processes sustaining this situation (including 'development') (see Odeh 2010).

8 It is in fact the assumed presence of this poverty that in recent years has started to draw attention to disability in the international sector, sustaining the raison d'être for large organisations such as Handicap International and Christian Blind Mission.

9 Over the centuries, fusions of beliefs, such as the indigenous Mayan religions blending Catholic, Christian and traditional beliefs and practices, have emerged, sometimes also as dynamics of resistance in colonial and neocolonial times.

10 These may not necessarily deny or stifle individual freedoms, especially when families and communities continue to ensure survival, including of their own disabled people.

References

Albrecht, G L, Seelman, K D and Bury, M (eds) 2001, *Handbook of disability studies*, Sage, Thousand Oaks.

Alkire, S 2006, 'Religion and development', in D Clark (ed.), *The Elgar companion to development studies*, Edward Elgar, Cheltenham, pp. 502–509.

Badiou, A 2002, *Ethics: an essay on the understanding of evil*, Verso, London.

Barnes, C and Mercer, G 2002, *Disability (key concepts)*, Blackwell, Oxford.

Barnes, C and Mercer, G 2010, *Exploring disability*, Polity Press, UK.

Barnes, C and Sheldon, A 2010, 'Disability, politics and poverty in a majority world context', *Disability and Society*, vol. 25, no. 7, pp. 771–782.

Barron, T and Ncube, J 2010, *Poverty and disability*, Leonard Cheshire International, London.

Berghs, M 2012, *War and embodied memory: becoming disabled in Sierra Leone*, Ashgate, UK and US.

Bird, S R 1996, 'Welcome to the men's club: homosociality and the maintenance of hegemonic masculinity', *Gender and Society*, vol. 10, no. 2, pp. 120–132.

Botello, N A 2005, 'The future that will not come: the eradication of poverty from the Mexican federal government's viewpoint (2000–2006)', in A Cimadamore, H Dean and J Siquiera (eds), *The poverty of the state*, CLASCO, Argentina, pp. 109–134.

Cutajar, J 2008, 'Knowledge and post-colonial pedagogy', *Mediterranean Journal of Educational Studies*, vol. 13, no. 2, pp. 27–47.

Davis, L J 2010, *The disability studies reader*, Routledge, New York and London.

Fanon, F 1963, *The wretched of the earth*, Grove Press, New York.

FAO 2008, 'Soaring food prices: facts, perspectives, impacts and actions required', paper presented at the High-Level Conference on World Food Security: The Challenges of Climate Change and Bioenergy, Rome, 3–5 June.

García Canclini, N 2005, *Hybrid cultures: strategies for entering and leaving modernity*, University of Minneapolis Press, Minneapolis.

Ghai, A 2002, 'Disability in the Indian context: post-colonial perspectives', in M Corker and T Shakespeare (eds), *Disability/postmodernity: embodying disability theory*, Continuum, London, pp. 88–100.

Grech, S 2009, 'Disability, poverty and development: critical reflections on the majority world debate', *Disability and Society*, vol. 24, no. 6, pp. 771–784.

Grech, S 2010, 'A space for "development": engaging social capital in reflecting on disability in the majority world', *Journal for Disability and International Development*, vol. 1, August, pp. 4–13.

Grech, S 2011, 'Recolonising debates or perpetuated coloniality? Decentring the spaces of disability, development and community in the global South', *International Journal of Inclusive Education*, vol. 15, no. 1, pp. 87–100.

Habashi, J 2005, 'Creating indigenous discourse: history, power, and imperialism in academia, Palestinian case', *Qualitative Inquiry*, vol. 11, no. 5, pp. 771–788.

IFAD 2011, *Rural poverty report 2011: new realities, new challenges*, IFAD, Rome.

Ingstad, B and Whyte, S R (eds) 2007, *Disability in local and global worlds*, University of California Press, Berkeley.

Livingston, J 2006, 'Insights from an African history of disability', *Radical History Review*, Winter, pp. 111–126.

Maclachlan, M and Swartz, L (eds) 2009, *Disability and international development: towards inclusive global health*, Springer, New York.

Meekosha, H 2011, 'Decolonizing disability: thinking and acting globally', *Disability and Society*, vol. 26, no. 6, pp. 667–682.

Miles, M 2000, 'High level baloney for third world disabled people', *Disability World*, vol. 5, October–December, accessed 19 March 2013, www.disabilityworld.org/10-12_00/news/baloney.htm.

Mkhize, N 2004, 'Psychology: an African perspective', in D Hook (ed.), *Critical psychology*, UCT Press, Lansdowne, pp. 24–52.

Mulligan, D and Gooding, K 2009, *The Millennium Development Goals and people with disabilities*, Sightsavers International, UK.

Narayan, D, Patel, R, Schafft, K, Rademacher, A and Koch-Schulte, S 2000, *Voices of the poor: can anyone hear us?*, Oxford University Press, Washington, DC.

Nederveen Pieterse, J 2001, 'Hybridity, so what? The anti-hybridity backlash and the riddles of recognition', *Theory, Culture & Society*, vol. 18, no. 2–3, pp. 219–245.

Odeh, L E 2010, 'A comparative analysis of global north and global south economies', *Journal of Sustainable Development in Africa*, vol. 12, no. 3, pp. 338–348.

Oliver, M 1996, *Understanding disability: from theory to practice*, Macmillan, Basingstoke.

Pfeiffer, D 2007, 'The disability studies paradigm', in P Devlieger, F Rusch and D Pfeiffer (eds), *Rethinking disability: the emergence of new definitions, concepts and communities*, Garant Publishers, Antwerp, pp. 95–110.

Pisani, M 2013, '"We are going to fix your vagina, just the way we like it": some reflections on the construction of [sub-Saharan] African female asylum seekers in Malta and their efforts to speak back', *Post Colonial Directions in Education*, vol. 2, no. 1, pp. 68–99.

Quijano, A 2008, 'Coloniality of power, eurocentrism, and social classification', in M Moraña, E Dussel and C A Jauregui (eds), *Coloniality at large: Latin America and the postcolonial debate*, Duke University Press, Durham, NC, pp. 181–224.

Said, E 1979, *Orientalism*, Vintage, New York.

Said, E 1993, *Culture and imperialism*, Vintage, New York.

Santos, B D 2009, 'A non-occcidental west? Learned ignorance and ecology of knowledge, theory', *Culture & Society*, vol. 26, no. 7–8, pp. 103–125.

Santos, B D 2012, 'Public spheres and epistemologies of the South', *Africa Development*, vol. XXXVII, pp. 43–67.

Satterthwaite, J 2008, 'Introduction', in J Satterthwaite, M Watts and H Piper (eds), *Talking truth, confronting power*, Trentham, London, pp. ix–xvii.

Siebers, T 2010, 'Disability and the theory of complex embodiment: for identity politics in a new register', in L J Davis (ed.), *The disability studies reader*, Routledge, New York and London, pp. 316–335.

Soldatic, K and Biyanwila, J 2010, 'Tsunami and the construction of disabled southern body', *Sephis e-magazine*, vol. 6, no. 3, pp. 75–84.

Stubbs, D 2008, 'Closing the gap: making the rights-based approach real for people with disabilities in the ASEAN region', paper prepared for International Council on Social Welfare (ICSW) South East Asia and Pacific Region (SEAP) ASEAN GO-NGO FORUM, Manila, December.

UNESCO 2010, *EFA global report 2010: reaching the marginalized*, UNESCO, Paris.

Weiss, M 2007, 'The chosen body and the rejection of disability in Israeli society', in B Ingstad and S R Whyte (eds), *Disability in local and global worlds*, University of California Press, Berkeley, pp. 107–127.

WHO 2009, 'Diarrhoeal disease: fact sheet N°330', accessed 6 February 2013, www.who.int/mediacentre/factsheets/fs330/en/index.html.

WHO 2010, *Trends in maternal mortality: 1990 to 2008*, WHO, Geneva.

WHO and World Bank 2011, *World report on disability*, WHO and World Bank, Washington, DC.

Whyte, S R and Ingstad, B 1995, 'Disability and culture: an overview', in B Ingstad and S R Whyte (eds), *Disability and culture*, University of California Press, Berkeley, pp. 3–32.

4 Accessible public space for the 'not obviously disabled'

Jeopardised selfhood in an era of welfare retraction

Alan Roulstone and Hannah Morgan

Background and context

The specific prompts for this chapter are changing and increasingly critical discourses of public space, participation and legitimacy and their implications for disabled people. Ironically these discourses, rather than view the problem as disabled people being excluded from public space, instead increasingly construct the problem, or at least a policy preoccupation, as disabled people being disengaged from public and economic space (Gregg, 2008). Not only do we see these discourses as negating policy objectives in making space and economic opportunity available, but also see the harsh content of these discourses such as 'shirkers and scroungers' (Briant *et al.*, 2011; Garthwaite, 2011), as de facto confirming 'sick and disabled' people's marginalisation. In that vein, we aim to explore the space between disabled people's self-perceptions, internalised and potentially jeopardised selfhoods, and the increasingly harsh welfare policy and media discourses, and most especially, for those who are presented as 'not genuinely disabled people'. In this sense we argue that enabling or disabling space has to be viewed as part physical, part social and part psychological phenomenon. We also contend that policy and political ideology as inscribed in public space are constitutive of the disabled and failed-disabled identity. Our work derives largely from developments in the UK, but we feel the neo-liberal dynamics that sit behind the increasing jeopardisation of space is likely to characterise other 'advanced' economies that have seen welfare growth and fiscal crises.

The material, physical and social basis of public space

Public space tends to be understood even within academic debates as a technical, physical measureable space, one characterised as external to the individual (Imrie and Kumar, 1998). Technologies similarly are often constructed as new technical means to afford or limit access to those environments (Gleeson, 1999). Policy constructions of space tend to equate the notion with access (BSI, 2005; Disability Rights Taskforce, 1999; DRC, 2000, 2002, 2004; ODPM, 2000). Even critical sociological accounts equate public space with the birth of the democratic principle and see its defining characteristics as *shared not owned*, a counter to bourgeois capitalism's tendency to translate social goods into marketable and privatised commodities (Habermas, 1989). Across the Western high-income economies at least, public space has been symbolic of greater social equity and decommodification, as for example in the public accessibility components of Roosevelt's New Deal (Leighninger, 1996). The involvement of the public in the design of public space also points up the shift historically towards the democratisation of space (Davidoff, 1965). From protesters from the large conurbations who undertook mass trespasses such as the Kinder Scout Trespass in 1932 as part of a campaign to open up private land for walkers (McKay, 2012) through to the recent mass global 'Occupy movement', occupying, reclaiming or subverting often restricted spaces has been a frequent tactic of many social movements. The disabled people's movement has frequently used public demonstrations, often in spaces of symbolic exclusion, to highlight the lack of access to public space that non-disabled people take for granted (Finkelstein, 1975; Zarb, 1995).

Disability studies and critical geography have also spawned a large literature on exclusive public space and the role of policy in making those environments more or less accessible (Clarke and George, 2005; Gleeson in Butler and Parr, 1999; Gray *et al.*, 2003; Hahn, 1986; Imrie and Kumar, 1998; Imrie and Wells, 1993). Perhaps closest to our own thinking on these issues is the work of Freund. In his article 'Bodies, disability and spaces' Freund (2001) makes the important point in stating:

> Here I stress sociomaterial space. The social organisation of space is not merely a place in which social interaction occurs, it structures such interaction. Congregating, avoiding people, movement and other practices constitute spatial patterns.

He further goes on to note:

> Sociomaterial space is not simply inert material – a configuration of asphalt and concrete – but exposes and structure's social life.
>
> (2001: 694)

Freund is useful here in going beyond a simple material 'bricks and mortar' account of public space. Indeed by using the notion of disability as 'bodies in space' he counters critiques of the social model as being disembodied (Freund, 2001). Even helpful recent discourses as to spatial inclusion do however have their limitations. Freund's work for example views spatial exclusion as increasingly rooted in auto-centred living and poor transport infrastructure. In this sense, the social and political interactions between bodies, self and environment, construct jeopardies too narrowly to capture recent events (Freund and Martin, 2001). Disability, health and embodiment are also rather taken for granted in this approach to [il]legitimate selfhood. As with Freund, our objective is to go beyond a physico-spatial construction of public space, or as the end product of urban planning/access policy, to broaden the analyses in a way that accounts for the overt politicisation of the public realm and, in turn, public space. In this sense space is constructed, maintained and shapes social relations. This is especially poignant where space constructs and maintains social distance and difference, as is often the case where disability and difference emerge into public spaces. There are literatures that apply notions of space and exclusions to an exploration of disability of course. For example, Dyck (1995) in her work 'Hidden geographies: the changing lifeworlds of women with disabilities', details the interaction of living with multiple sclerosis and the broader social, policy and environmental shaping of access, and notes:

> The majority of women were found to experience shrinking social and geographical worlds which rendered their lives increasingly hidden from view as patterns of social interaction changed and use of public space diminished.
>
> (1995: 307)

The focus of Dyck's study on the spatio-temporal settings of the women's everyday lives reveals:

> an interplay of biomedical discourse, policy structures, sociocultural norms and local sets of social relations that shape the strategies women used in re/constructing their lives. Participants showed a diversity of responses, but these were all characterized by a restructuring of home and neighbourhood space, a reordering of personal relationships and increasing interpenetration of the public sphere in their private lives. The findings suggest that attention to the body in its geographical as well as social context provides an avenue for investigating the links between subjective experience and the broader social relations and processes which shape the illness experience.
>
> (Dyck, 1995: 1)

Dyck's work is extremely helpful in aiding a socially and policy located notion of gendered space; however policy discourses are broadly inscribed via local influences and practices. Policy is merely one, albeit important, facet of Dyck's work. Perhaps closest to our construction and connection between disability and space is the work of Kitchin. Kitchin, in his article '"Out of place", "knowing one's place": space, power and the exclusion of disabled people', notes:

> space, as well as time, is instrumental in reproducing and sustaining disablist practices. Disability has distinct spatialities that work to exclude and oppress disabled people. Spaces are currently organised to keep disabled people 'in their place' and 'written' to convey to disabled people that they are 'out of place' ... As a result, forms of oppression and their reproduction within ideologies leads to distinct spatialities with the creation of landscapes of exclusion, the boundaries of which are reinforced through a combination of the popularising of cultural representations and the creation of myths.
>
> (Kitchin, 1998: 351)

Changing policy and remoralised corporeal economies

Space, or public space to be precise, is then more than the sum of physical, technological space, but potent psycho-social environments created by public discourses that need to be understood if we are to understand disabling/enabling space. This is especially true where an impairment is 'hidden', contested or fluctuating. The increasingly political emphasis on sifting the 'real' disabled people from the army of 'malingering opportunists' (HM Government, 2012) ignores the complex relationship between the individual, the environment and the moral economy of contemporary competitive society (Soldatic and Meekosha, 2012). Such mainstream policy constructions ignore medical, welfare and wider social constructions of just who counts as disabled. In trying to remoralise, to forcibly reintegrate those reconstructed in policy terms as 'faux' disabled people, we argue policy and public spaces paradoxically make such reintegration less rather than more likely (Roulstone and Prideaux, 2012). Of note, even key architects of the conditionality regime that underpins welfare and disability benefit reforms have now voiced their concern as to the harshness and levels of sophistication of the reassessment processes (Gregg, 2012). Recent official reports also point to national and governmental concerns over those reforms (Harrington, 2012; National Audit Office, 2012).

The debate as to who is, or is not, disabled has often been constructed using crude policy and representational (media) binaries (Briant *et al.*, 2011), ones that assume disability is fixed, static, knowable and easily measured. Disability, unlike race, sex/gender, age and genetic profile, cannot of course be viewed unproblematically. Disabled people can feel they are genuinely disabled in one definition and context and not another. They may feel they are chronically ill but not disabled, or disabled but not sick (deWolfe, 2002, 2012). In this sense, we wish to problematise space and acceptance/jeopardy to think about space as a contested terrain, both imagined and real, where lives are constructed as more or less acceptable in a new corporeal (bodily) economy. This new corporeal economy, one arguably driven by the retraction of the welfare state, has led to a number of major jeopardies, especially for those people who do not fit stereotyped images of disability (Boyd, 2012).

The social costs of such binary remoralisations are arguably not simply the potential loss of welfare, but, drawing on the valuable work of Thomas (1999) and Reeve's (2002) notion of psycho-emotional disablism, we can see the psycho-social costs of being deemed unfit for the new corporeal economy of space. According to Reeve for example, psycho-emotional disablism is the result of continued negative constructions and interactions which in turn create psycho-emotional barriers to future opportunity. In this context, barriers to *being* sit alongside and can be as powerful as barriers to *doing*, and have the potential to be more pervasive, persistent and disabling. Drawing on Reeve and Thomas' work then, there are likely to be emotional costs for some disabled people in 'moving through space' or failing to occupy economic space, even if through no fault of their own (Reeve, 2008). As we suggest below, the public realm may well have become much harsher, much more judgemental, as to who counts as legitimately disabled, and just who 'belongs'. Experience of those with hidden impairments and who may experience pain and fatigue are especially important here. The already medically contested physical or psychological condition also enters an increasingly socially contested space where hidden or unseen impairment may sit badly with new policy constructions of desert and eligibility (Garthwaite *et al.*, 2013). Psycho-social notions of disability can be defined as: the result of the interplay of physical, institutional, political and interpersonal constructions of 'desirable states'. Here, space is synonymous with 'locations' which welcome, exclude or *other* (Butler, 1990) disabled people. In this sense, space can be an object, a process, a project, an existential sense of belonging/exclusion.

Policy spaces and the changing environment for jeopardised selves

To the casual observer, the realm of say disability policy, interpreted as welfare and social care policy, and that of access and anti-discrimination policy, sit in very different policy and spatial locations and have not been in meaningful dialogue. Indeed, the idea that certain policy developments might negate others seems anathema to mainstream policy analyses. However it could be argued that emphasising fair and reasonable treatment in anti-discrimination policy (Disability Rights Taskforce, 1999) alongside increasingly harsh statements about disability welfare dependency (HM Government, 2012) helps unravel any potentially more progressive disability policy developments. Of note the failure to enforce key aspects of the Disability Discrimination Act (DDA) (1995) and the DDA Amendment Act (2005) leaves many barriers in place (Roberts *et al.*, 2004) or perversely can lead to the assumption that barriers have already been removed. The attachment of welfare dependency to sick and disabled people had not been a characteristic of the welfare state or wider welfare discourse from 1945 to 1997 (Roulstone and Prideaux, 2012). The exact causes of a hardening of rhetoric and the growing 'link' between sickness/disability and dependency are fiercely debated (Connor, 2010; Deacon and Patrick, 2011; Garthwaite, 2011; Hirst, 2007), however a careful analyses of the changing rhetoric and detail of policy reform makes cost-savings and the avoiding of a growing welfare/social care budget clear explanatory favourites (Duncan-Smith, 2012a).

The general tenor of welfare reform was established by the New Labour government from 1997 (Prideaux, 2005); however the rhetoric has hardened yet further with the accession of the British Coalition government (merger of British right and centrist parties) in what might be seen as a consolidation of anti-welfarist and anti-dependency thinking. The following from the newly installed Chancellor George Osborne makes clear their resolve in battling a welfare system that is viewed as 'out of control':

> I want to support the person who leaves their house at six or seven in the morning, goes out and does perhaps a low-paid job in order to provide for

their family and is incredibly frustrated when they see on the other side of the street the blinds pulled down and someone sitting there and living on out-of-work benefits.

(Osbourne, 2010)

Public and economic space have here become the focus of increased scrutiny and top-down discourse in a manner that affords little right to reply for those affected. The stridency and the power of these messages arguably creates the broad backdrop of jeopardised public space for those unable or unwilling to work. Both the system of welfare and those whose behaviour has been distorted by welfarism is clear in the following assertion from the incoming Secretary of State for Work and Pensions which is unambiguous in its use of derogatory and disablist language:

the benefits system is 'bust' and carries such disincentives to work that many people on benefits regard those who enter employment as 'bloody morons'.

(Duncan Smith, 2010)

Such rhetoric has not however, at least since the days of the English Poor Law (1601, 1834) (Boyer, 1990; Topliss, 1975), connected disability, frailty, sickness and bodily difficulty (or faux versions of these) with such harsh welfare narratives. In fact a founding characteristic of the early welfare system was its concern for those who could not make a contribution via taxation or national insurance as they were too ill or faced too many barriers gaining access to production (as workers) and often consumption spaces (as consumers). Concern to help those who were outside the economic system of advanced capitalism also sat beneath the development of key facets of the welfare state, most notably the National Health Service (Topliss, 1975). Whether one sees this as perpetuating the view that disabled people should be cared for or given what the state felt was best (paternalism) is a moot point. However, there is risk in both right-ideology and a productivist form of disability studies (see Abberley, 1999) that they might both inadvertently overlook those who face the greatest social barriers, that is, sickness and impairment effects. Unlike the English Poor Law there are many sick and disabled people who cannot work but who are being told they can work (Garthwaite *et al.*, 2013) in the new corporeal economy of welfare reform. Certainly the recent coupling of welfare reform with sickness and disability is perhaps the most important development of the last 60 years of UK social policy (Roulstone and Prideaux, 2012). The certainty of the cause, response and justification of welfare reform and the inclusion of disability/sickness is made clear in the following statement by the UK prime minister:

Politicians often overcomplicate their analysis, but actually, it's quite simple. It comes back to responsibility. When the welfare system was born, there was what we might call a collective culture of responsibility. More than today, people's self-image was not just about their personal status or success it was measured out by what sort of citizen they were; whether they did the decent thing ... That meant that a standardised system of sickness and out-of-work benefits – with limited conditions – was effective. It reached the people who needed that support, and not those who didn't, in part because fiddling the system would have brought not just public outcry but private shame. In other words, personal responsibility acted as a brake on abuse of the system. And because the ethos of self-betterment was more wide-spread, the system supported aspiration rather than discouraging it.

(Cameron, 2011)

The romanticising of a bygone welfare age and system of personal responsibility forms the basis of an ideological justification of the need for change. It is assumed that many people jumped on the sickness and disability bandwagon as a way to avoid paid work. The growth in benefits is attributed to worklessness and loss of citizen-impulse and not due to illness, impairment and barriers. Additionally, the argument is put that the disability benefits system is too easily manipulated due to vagaries in the system itself, for example the Disability Living Allowance (extra costs benefit) (DLA) system:

A lot of that is down to the way the benefit [DLA] was structured so that it was very loosely defined.

(Duncan Smith, 2012b)

Both the presentation of a 'golden age' of welfare and the decline into dependency are each complementary but highly questionable in factual terms (Garthwaite, 2011). Indeed a veritable flood of critique, counter-evidence and activism has arisen to attempt to challenge this welfare reform project. However there is evidence of real, negative and possibly enduring hardship and divisiveness for many sick and disabled people (National Audit Office, 2012). The public domain, one where we can claim and reaffirm our sense of belonging, has arguably become a terrain of conflict and hostility towards the so-called 'not genuinely disabled' as the media portrayal and evidence of hate crime below attests. This is in spite of the acknowledgement that key components of welfare reform, such as alleged fraud, is now acknowledged by the UK government to be overstated:

The truth is quite a lot of what we here politically term constantly as fraud is often complexity error, which is very easy for us to then say this is fraud and people feel quite stigmatised by that ... the truth is quite a lot is nothing to do with them, it's the system itself. It simply means they didn't understand what they were meant to be doing and now they are apparently committing fraud and a lot of them didn't know that was the case.

(Duncan Smith, 2011)

The officially acknowledged fraud rate for disability benefits is 1.5 per cent (National Audit Office, 2009), whilst the real reasons for DLA growth is mostly to do with ageing on DLA with the growth of the over-65 claimant count and an increase in children surviving previously deadly impairments (DWP, 2012a). These are images far from that of a burgeoning mass of scroungers with little or no sickness or impairment. Of note this is not the first time such policy claims of growth via fraud have bedevilled the disability benefits system, an earlier moral panic about DLA had taken place in 1998, whilst the final analyses led to similar paucity of evidence of fraud as a rather apologetic ministerial response to a parliamentary select committee made clear back in 1998:

> I am not quite sure what you mean by robust. In terms of DLA [Disability Living Allowance], it is extremely difficult to identify quite whether it is fraud … I do think it is about correctness and we are sure that there is a high level of incorrectness there.
>
> (UK Parliament, 1998)

Despite the evidence of the thinness of argument behind the detail of welfare reform, the impact on sick and disabled is very real. Public space becomes saturated with daily stories of disability fraud and scrounging (Briant *et al.*, 2011). Many of the stories afford little or no right to reply, many of the people highlighted have impairments but have been caught functioning in ways that are not congruent with disability benefit claims. This is noteworthy as the need to emphasise everything you cannot do (as opposed to objective medical assessments) characterises disability benefit claim processes (Beatty *et al.*, 2009). The impact for many is a state of fear and apathy that whatever they say or do, the state will, they believe, arbitrarily decide on whether a person is 'legitimately' disabled or not (Soldatic, 2013). For example the recent target to get 0.5 million claimants off DLA (an extra costs benefit) makes clear that a number of disabled people who had been medically accredited to be 'disabled for life' would possibly be deemed not disabled enough for the new benefit – Personal Independence Payment (PIP) (Deacon and Patrick, 2011).

There is clear evidence that there has been a significant shift in the focus and tenor of media coverage of disability. In their recent report, *Bad news for disabled people: how the newspapers are reporting disability*, Briant *et al.* (2011) found there had been an increase of over 30 per cent in the number of articles concerned with disability between 2004–5 and 2010–1. Whilst this increase is perhaps unsurprising given the growing awareness of disabled people in a range of forums and particularly as customers/consumers (ODI, 2012), what is of concern is the emphasis and tone of this coverage, much of which echoes the politicised and vitriolic nature of speeches by key government ministers we cite above. In particular there has been the presentation of disability status as a privileged and mis-used option for the 'faux' disabled.

> There has been a significantly increased use of pejorative language to describe disabled people, including suggestions that life on incapacity benefit had become a 'Lifestyle Choice'.
>
> (Briant *et al.*, 2011: 5)

This is well illustrated by the following diatribe by a well-known columnist in which he tastelessly suggests 'pretending' to be disabled enough to secure benefits is both fashionable and easy:

> My New Year's resolution for 2012 was to become disabled. Nothing too serious, maybe just a bit of a bad back or one of those newly invented illnesses which make you a bit peaky for decades – fibromyalgia or M.E … And being disabled is incredibly fashionable. The number of people who claim to be disabled has doubled in the past ten years … It has become easier to claim those benefits, partly as a consequence of the disablement charities who, out of their own self-interest, insist that an ever-greater proportion of the population is disabled … I think we should all pretend to be disabled for a month or so, claim benefits and hope this persuades the authorities to sort out the mess.
>
> (Liddle, 2012)

The piece also echoes the report finding that those with 'hidden' or socially 'unsympathetic' conditions were more likely to be described as 'undeserving' (11) whilst the attitudes of participants in the accompanying focus groups were summed up as 'disabled people are not fraudsters and fraudsters are not disabled people' (13) with clear implications for those who are either 'not-obviously' disabled or perceived not to be 'disabled enough'.

Moreover the report noted that claims in the media, and much repeated elsewhere, about extremely high levels of disability benefit fraud were 'made overwhelmingly without evidence' (Briant *et al.*, 2011: 12) and without a concurrent acknowledgement of the officially collated figures that document extremely low levels of fraud: 0.3 per cent for Incapacity Benefit and 0.5 per cent for DLA (DWP, 2012b: 14).

A particular feature of the coverage highlighted by the report was the way in which the explanations for benefit claims were personalised and pathologised as these fairly representative tweets by @thisisamy suggest:

> Collectively, this government & certain media have made me feel that I am at fault for having a disability. That I choose it.
>
> (@thisisamy, 2013a)

> As a disabled person, I do feel persecuted & singled out.
>
> (@thisisamy, 2013b)

This is part of a much wider discourse about all those who claim benefits captured in the phrase 'scroungers or strivers' that implies a false dichotomy between those who claim benefits and those in work that fails to acknowledge the barriers that many disabled people face in accessing the labour market or that benefits like the DLA enable significant numbers of disabled people to work. What is apparent from this analysis is that political and media discourses around disability and ('faux') disabled people have been effective in influencing popular perceptions. As Tyler notes social media is increasingly used to 'harden public opinion into consent' and that the 'symbolic violence' witnessed there 'is converted into forms of material violence that are embodied and lived' (2013: 211–12). This can be experienced as direct disablism, in acts of naked aggression and violence targeting disabled people or perhaps more invidiously as Reeve suggests in her chapter as indirect psycho-emotional disablism whereby disabled people's experiences of moving through public space are uncomfortable and inhospitable.

Responses to jeopardised space and demonised selfhood

Despite the harshness of policy space and the propagation of myriad stories about scrounging and faked disability, it would be wrong to portray disabled people as willing victims of these discourses and as lacking agency (Findlay-Williams, 2011). However the truly destructive development aspects of these new policy and public constructions is that no one quite knows *who* it is that deviates from acceptable definitions of disability and claimancy. Indeed a key aspect of jeopardised public space is that we cannot often know who has an impairment, who experiences pain, fatigue and social barriers. Apart from disabled people who are obviously akin to stereotypes of disabled people – wheelchair users, people with learning difficulties – the 'obviously' different; the preponderance of people with state accredited impairments have often unseen musculo-skeletal, heart, chest or neurological challenges (Department of Health, 2012). In fact, a number of people will be what might be called 'sick disabled' and have hard-to-manage and frequently fluctuating impairments/illnesses. These disabled people may arguably be at risk of being overlooked by new policy discourses built on visible stereotypes and have also been largely overlooked by disability studies where the emphasis has often been on playing down pain, fatigue and impairment effects (Mont, 2007).

Because we often do not know who counts in a public context such spaces and equivalent policy spaces arguably draw on hunches, convictions, clues and revelatory news stories which unearth the 'truth' about impairment or pretence at a disability status. The result is akin to a form of mutual public paranoia, that any one individual may be a benefit cheat and be affecting disability status, whilst for sick and disabled people, some of whom may have been reluctant to take on a disabled identity due to fear of stigma, may now fear being found 'not disabled' or not disabled enough to meet the threshold of state-accredited impairment. Frequently this is the result of changes to eligibility criteria rather than a change in a condition or level of impairment which further blurs the distinction between genuine and faux disabled people (Grover and Soldatic, 2013). As we discuss above public perception of a reducing number of claimants is that individuals have withdrawn from claiming benefits to avoid being 'found out' rather than the result of heightened eligibility criteria and a harsh and dehumanising assessment process. Furthermore, there has been a disassociation in much popular discourse of the perceived 'perks' disabled people enjoy, such as the blue badge parking scheme or DLA.

These are new developments and the closest parallels in recent history are the psycho-dynamics of authoritarian states where unorthodox or unapproved thoughts and behaviours lead to informing and often very severe sanctions (Fitzpatrick, 1999). These ideas are not confined to policy and ideological pronouncements but it can be argued begin to pervade public space as powerful dynamics and behavioural forces which make life hugely conditional and fearful for many disabled people (Garthwaite, 2011). The recent shift from DLA to PIPs is a case in point. The higher rate threshold to establish a claimant's rights to have their independence supported is being reset to a point where a disabled person cannot walk more than 20 metres without risk of harm, danger or severe discomfort (Dunt, 2013). Many disabled people are querying how such a stipulation can form the basis of an independence-driven agenda. For example for those that can walk 50 metres (the previous threshold) their ready access to independence and support is stopped off, whilst those 'successful' in claiming higher rate PIP may be likely to fear being seen walking more than that distance (Dunt, 2013). Here then is an inadvertent extension of possible stigma and fear for those who have more obvious and visible impairments. Whether one takes the example of the person with an unseen impairment fearing exposure or an individual with a visible impairment afraid to be seen walking more than 20 metres, new welfare discourses will undoubtedly lead to increasingly jeopardised identities in public space.

What then of the impact of these changes to public space? There are many manifestations of disabled people's fears, for brevity, the following are typical of many thousands of statements that populate blogs and e-bulletins in 2013:

> I don't think about what might happen to me if the government's proposed threats/changes actually materialise. I firmly push it to the back of my mind, burying it as deep as I can so not to be overwhelmed by panic and fear about a situation I can do nothing about … The kind of fear that is hard to describe. The type that sits, deep in the pit of your stomach and travels up in to your throat where if you let it will clench it's fist and take hold starving you of breath.
>
> (Ouch! web blog, 2008)

The following is a parent's letter to the editor of a well-known newspaper which supports an eye hospital wing where their daughter is being treated, whilst championing the newspaper editor's alarmist and wildly inaccurate editorials on disability scrounging. The parent of the disabled child notes the irony of this apparent incongruity of approach:

> Just over a year ago, my daughter Eve, then aged three, was diagnosed with chronic uveitis, an inflammation of the eyes that can cause blindness … I was shocked to discover she had no vision in one eye and the other was deteriorating … But it is another of your business interests that I find more difficult to square with your support for Moorfields [eye hospital]: the Daily Express – and its relentless war on sick and disabled benefit claimants. Recent front page stories include:

75% on sick are skiving – benefit cheats are taking us to the cleaners

Blitz on Britain's benefits madness – scroungers use 500 scams to grab your cash

Blitz on benefits: 887,000 fiddlers exposed

So here's a novel idea. The next time a DWP briefing comes your way, instead of repeating it, scrutinise it. In these austere times it needn't cost your newsroom extra cash. The Express recently complained that, according to DWP figures, 'spots, indigestion and sunburn' were among the reasons claimants received benefit, while the Daily Mail mocked other ailments such as 'diarrhoea' and 'nail disorders'. But a glance at the DWP survey's footnotes would have revealed that these conditions were not necessarily the reason benefits were given.

(Singer, 2011)

Whilst one disabled person is using artistic expression to convey the degree to which a climate of fear places some disabled people in a twilight world: one where they are afraid to be seen doing anything that might be construed as at odds with benefit criteria. This is of course some distance from the objectives of independence and choice at the heart of wider disability policy reforms of the 1990s:

For some months, I have lain low for fear of being penalised, but instead of letting fear determine who I am, I'd rather stare it in the face … I want to make a twilight existence visible, but more than that, I want to show that what many people see as contradiction – what they describe as fraud – is only the complexity of real life.

(Pring, 2011)

Conclusion: rights, wrongs and jeopardised public space

From the outset we have argued that space, or public space to be precise, is more than the sum of physical, technological space – potent psycho-social environments created by public discourses need to be understood if we are to understand disabling/enabling space. What can we glean from the above exploration of media portrayal, new constructions of welfare dependency, behavioural distortions 'wrought' by the welfare state and our understanding of public space?

It is probably best to compare an idealised model of inclusion and belonging and to place that in parallel to the environment that is being (inadvertently or deliberately?) created by recent discourses on welfare and disability. The following aims to represent the difference between an idealised picture of citizenship by drawing on key principles of the UN Convention on the Rights of Disabled People (UN, 2006) whilst contrasting these with the increasingly jeopardised state that many disabled people find themselves in. Although the Convention does not operationalise rights to inclusive and humane spaces beyond an anti-discrimination legal construction of access, the spirit of the Convention captures well a range of measures of enabled citizenship that many disabled people would aspire to (see Table 4.1).

Table 4.1 Public space, inclusion and jeopardy: a comparison with the UN Convention precepts (excerpted) (UN, 2006, www.un.org/disabilities/convention/conventionfull. shtml).

UN Convention Precepts	Risk that Inhere in Stigmatising Policy
Dignity, autonomy, independence	Jeopardised selfhoods, enforced behavioural norms
Full and effective participation and inclusion	Fear of participation, hostile public spaces in society; psycho-social exclusion
Respect for difference	Propagated fear of difference, hatred of difference
Humanity and diversity	Uncertainty, stigmatising or unseen or 'hidden' impairment
Equality of opportunity	Engrain and reinforce disablism, fear of disability, fear of being in public, fear of assault

The above makes clear the hardening rhetoric around disability and welfare dependency. Academic analyses to date have attempted to explore the nature, accuracy and purpose of such changing rhetoric. In this chapter we have entered into a new line of analysis in looking at the impact of these changing discourses on constructions of disability, legitimacy and selfhood. We argue that spaces are increasingly jeopardised for many disabled people. Living lives of fulfilment, rights and choices has been made harder in this climate. Only the future will tell us the longer-term impact of such new jeopardies.

References

Abberley, P 1999, 'The significance of work for the citizenship of disabled people', paper presented at University College Dublin, 15 April, accessed 13 May 2013, http:// disability-studies.leeds.ac.uk/files/library/Abberley-sigofwork.pdf.

@thisisamy 2013a, 'Collectively, this government & certain media have made me feel that I am at fault for having a disability. That I choose it', #beddingout 11 April, accessed 7 May 2013, https://twitter.com/thisisamy_/status/322382656119652352.

@thisisamy 2013b, '@lisapeacefrench yes you're right. As a disabled person, I do feel persecuted & singled out', #beddingout 13 April, accessed 7 May 2013, https://twitter. com/thisisamy_/status/322386699428704256.

Beatty, C, Fothergill, S and Platts-Fowler, D 2009, 'DLA claimants – a new assessment: the characteristics and aspirations of the Incapacity Benefit claimants who receive Disability Living Allowance', *DWP Research Report No 585*, DWP, Norwich.

Boyd, V 2012, 'Are some disabilities more equal than others? Conceptualising fluctuating or recurring impairments within contemporary legislation and practice', *Disability and Society*, vol. 27, no. 4, pp. 459–469.

Boyer, G 1990, *An economic history of the English poor law, 1750–1850*, Cambridge University Press, Cambridge.

Briant, B, Watson, N and Philo, G 2011, *Bad news for disabled people: how the newspapers are reporting disability*, Inclusion London and Glasgow University.

British Standards Institution (BSI) 2005, *BS7000-6: Design management systems: managing inclusive design*, BSI, London.

Butler, J 1990, *Gender trouble: feminism and the subversion of identity*, Routledge, New York.

Butler, R and Parr, H (eds) 1999, *Mind and body spaces: geographies of illness, impairment, and disability (critical geographies)*, Routledge, New York.

Cameron, D 2011, *Prime Minister – speech on Welfare Reform Bill*, 17 February, accessed 13 April 2013, www.number10.gov.uk/news/pms-speech-on-welfare-reform-bill/.

Clarke, P and George, L K 2005, 'The role of the built environment in the disablement process', *American Journal of Public Health*, vol. 95, no. 11, pp. 1933–1939.

Connor, S 2010, 'Promoting "employability": the changing subject of *Welfare* reform in the UK', *Critical Discourse Analysis*, vol. 7, no. 1, pp. 41–45.

Davidoff, P 1965, 'Advocacy and pluralism in planning', *Journal of the American Institute of Planners*, vol. 31, no. 4, pp. 331–337.

Deacon, A and Patrick, R 2011, 'A new welfare settlement? The Coalition government and welfare-to-work', in H Bochel (ed.), *The conservative party and social policy*, The Policy Press, Bristol, pp. 161–179.

deWolfe, P 2002, 'Private tragedy in social context? Reflections on disability, illness and suffering', *Disability and Society*, vol. 17, no. 3, pp. 255–267.

deWolfe, P 2012, 'Reaping the benefits of sickness? Long-term illness and the experience of welfare claims', *Disability and Society*, vol. 27, no. 5, pp. 617–630.

Department of Health 2012, *Third edition of long term conditions compendium*, DoH, London.

Department for Work and Pensions (DWP) 2012a, *DWP information, governance and security, work and pensions longitudinal study: time series DLA claimants by age*, accessed 13 May 2013, www.gov.uk/government/news/statistical-update-disability-living-allowance-claims.

Department for Work and Pensions (DWP) 2012b, *Fraud and error in the benefit system: 2010/11 estimates (Great Britain)*, accessed 12 May 2013, http://research.dwp.gov.uk/asd/asd2/fem/fem_apr10_mar11.pdf.

Disability Rights Commission (DRC) 2000, *Making access to goods and services easier for disabled customers: a practical guide for small businesses and other small service providers*, DRC, Manchester.

Disability Rights Commission (DRC) 2002, *Code of practice. Rights of access. Goods, facilities, services and premises*, The Stationery Office, London.

Disability Rights Commission (DRC) 2004, *Access statements: achieving an inclusive environment by ensuring continuity throughout the planning, design and management of buildings and spaces*, DRC, Stratford-upon-Avon.

Disability Rights Taskforce 1999, *From exclusion to inclusion; a report of the Disability Rights Task Force on Civil Rights for Disabled People*, DRC Legacy Document, accessed 13 April 2013, www.leeds.ac.uk/disabilitystudies/archiveuk/disability%20rights%20task%20force/From%20exclusion%20to%20inclusion.pdf.

Duncan-Smith, I 2010, 'Interview', *Guardian*, 26 May.

Duncan-Smith, I 2011, *Evidence to the Work and Pensions Select Committee*, 10 February UK Parliament.

Duncan-Smith, I 2012a, *Welfare reforms realised*, DWP Press Release, 8 March, accessed 13 April 2013, www.dwp.gov.uk/newsroom/press-releases/2012/mar-2012/dwp023-12.shtml.

Duncan Smith, I 2012b, 'Article on welfare reform', *Telegraph*, 14 May.

Dunt, I 2013, 'The tyranny of the 20 metre test: Atos presides over hated change in disability benefit', *Politics.Co.UK*, 8 April, accessed 13 April 2013, www.politics.co.uk/news/2013/04/08/the-tyranny-of-the-20-metre-test-atos-presides-over-hated-ch.

Dyck, I 1995, 'Hidden geographies: the changing lifeworlds of women with disabilities', *Social Science and Medicine*, vol. 40, no. 3, pp. 307–320.

Findlay-Williams, R 2011, 'Lifting the lid on disabled people against cuts', *Disability and Society*, vol. 26, no. 6, pp. 773–778.

Finkelstein, V 1975, 'Phase 2: discovering the person in "Disability" and "Rehabilitation"', *Magic Carpet*, vol. 27, no. 1, pp. 31–38.

Fitzpatrick, S 1999, *Everyday Stalinism: ordinary life in extraordinary times: Soviet Russia in the 1930s*, Oxford University Press, Oxford.

Freund, P 2001, 'Bodies, disability and spaces: the social model and disabling spatial organisations', *Disability and Society*, vol. 16, no. 5, pp. 689–706.

Freund, P and Martin, G 2001, 'Moving bodies: injury, dis-ease and the social organization of space', *Critical Public Health*, vol. 11, no. 3, pp. 203–214.

Garthwaite, K 2011, '"The language of shirkers and scroungers?" Talking about illness, disability and coalition welfare reform', *Disability and Society*, vol. 26, no. 3, May, pp. 369–372.

Garthwaite, K, Warren, J and Bambra, C 2013, '"The unwilling and the unwell"? Exploring stakeholders' perceptions of working with long term sickness benefits recipients', *Disability and Society*, 28(8), pp. 1104–1117.

Gleeson, B 1999, *Geographies of disability*, Routledge, London.

Gray, D B, Gould, M and Bickenbach, J E 2003, 'Environmental barriers and disability', *Journal of Architecture and Planning Research*, vol. 20, pp. 29–37.

Gregg, P 2008, *Realising potential: a vision for personalised conditionality and support,* An independent report to the Department for Work and Pensions, DWP, London.

Gregg, P 2012, 'New ideas for disability, employment and welfare reform', key note lecture at Hardest Hit Event, Leeds University, UK, 20 September.

Grover, C and Soldatic, K 2013, 'Neoliberal restructuring, disabled people and social (in)security in Australia and Britain', *Scandinavian Journal of Disability Research*, 15(3), pp. 216–232.

Habermas, J 1989, *The structural transformation of the public sphere: an inquiry into a category of bourgeois society*, MIT Press, Cambridge, MA.

Hahn, H 1986, 'Disability and the urban environment: a perspective on Los Angeles', *Environment and Planning D: Society and Space*, vol. 4, pp. 273–288.

Harrington, M 2012, *An independent review of the work capability assessment – year three*, November, The Stationery Office, London.

Hirst, K 2007, *Working welfare*, Adam Smith Institute, London.

HM Government 2012, *Statute: Welfare Reform Act*, accessed 13 April 2013, www.services.parliament.uk/bills/2010–11/welfarereform.html.

Imrie, R F and Kumar, M 1998, 'Focusing on disability and access in the built environment', *Disability and Society*, vol. 13, pp. 357–374.

Imrie, R and Wells, P 1993, 'Disablism, planning, and the built environment', *Environment and Planning C: Government and Policy*, vol. 11, no. 2, pp. 213–231.

Kitchin, R M 1998, '"Out of place", "knowing one's place": towards a spatialised theory of disability and social exclusion', *Disability and Society*, vol. 13, no. 3, pp. 343–356.

Leighninger, R D 1996, 'Cultural infrastructure: the legacy of new deal public space', *Journal of Architectural Education*, vol. 49, no. 4, pp. 226–236.

Liddle, R 2012, '"Pretend disabled" really ARE sick', *Sun*, 26 January.

McKay, S 2012, *Ramble on: the story of our love for walking*, Harper Collins, London.

Mont, D 2007, *Measuring disability prevalence*, Washington, DC, World Bank (SP Discussion Paper No.0706), accessed 13 April 2013, http://siteresources.worldbank.org/DISABILITY/Resources/Data/MontPrevalence.pdf.

National Audit Office 2009, Department for Work and Pensions: Resource Account 2009–10, NAO, London, accessed 13 May 2013, www.nao.org.uk/wp-content/uploads/2010/07/dwp_accounts_0910.pdf.

National Audit Office 2012, *A commentary for the Committee Of Public Accounts On The Work Programme, outcome statistics report by The Comptroller and Auditor General*, Hc 832session 2012-13,13 December, NAO, London.

Office of the Deputy Prime Minister (ODPM) 2000, *Building regulations: part M*, The Stationery Office, London.

Office for Disability Issues (ODI) 2012, *Growing your customer base to include disabled people: a guide for businesses*, accessed 12 May 2013, http://odi.dwp.gov.uk/docs/idp/Growing-your-customer-base-to-include-disabled-people.pdf.

Ouch! 2008, *Who is afraid of welfare reform? Guest Post by The Goldfish*, 31 March, accessed 23 May 2013, www.bbc.co.uk/blogs/ouch/2008/03/whos_afraid_of_welfare_reform.html.

Osbourne, G. (2010) Pre-budget Discussion of Welfare Reform, BBC Andrew Marr Show, June 19 (http://news.bbc.co.uk/1/hi/programmes/andrew_marr_show/8750301.stm).

Prideaux, S 2005, *Not so new Labour: a sociological critique of new Labour's policy and practice*, Policy Press, Bristol.

Pring, J 2011, 'Crow will make the private public in defence of her bed life', 28 March, accessed 13 April 2013, http://disabilitynewsservice.com/2013/03/crow-will-make-the-private-public-in-defence-of-her-bed-life/.

Reeve, D 2002, 'Negotiating psycho-emotional dimensions of disability and their influence on identity constructions', *Disability and Society*, vol. 17, no. 5, pp. 493–508.

Reeve, D 2008, 'Negotiating disability in everyday life: the experience of psycho-emotional disablism', PhD thesis, Lancaster University

Roberts, S, Heaver, C, Hill, C, Rennison, J, Stafford, B, Howat, N, Kelly, G, Krishnan, S, Tapp, P and Thomas, A 2004, *Disability in the workplace: employers' and service providers' responses to the Disability Discrimination Act in 2003 and preparation for the 2004 changes*, DWP, London.

Roulstone, A and Prideaux, S 2012, *Understanding disability policy*, Policy Press, Bristol.

Singer, C 2011, *Stop demonising disabled claimants: an open letter to Richard Desmond*, 9 May, accessed 13 April 2013, http://falseeconomy.org.uk/blog/stop-demonising-disabled-claimants-open-letter-richard-desmond.

Soldatic, K 2013, 'Appointment time: disability and neoliberal workfare temporalities', *Critical Sociology*, vol. 39, no. 3, pp. 405–419.

Soldatic, K and Meekosha, H 2012, 'The place of disgust: disability, class and gender in spaces of workfare', *Societies*, vol. 2, no. 3, pp. 139–156.

Thomas, C 1999, *Female forms: experiencing and understanding disability*, Open University Press, Buckingham.

Topliss, E 1975, *Provision for the disabled*, 2nd edn, Blackwell/Martin Robertson, Oxford.

Tyler, I 2013, *Revolting subjects: social abjection and resistance in neoliberal Britain*, Zed Books, London.

UK Parliament 1998, *Public Accounts Committee: examination of witnesses (questions 80 – 99)*, 18 February, accessed 13 April 2013, www.publications.parliament.uk/pa/cm199798/cmselect/cmpubacc/570/8021806.htm.

United Nations (UN) 2006, Convention on the Rights of Persons with Disabilities [CRPD] G.A. Res. 61/106, U.N. Doc. A/61/611, 13 December, www.un.org/esa/socdev/enable/rights/convtexte.htm.

Zarb, G 1995, *Removing disabling barriers*, Policy Studies Institute, London.

5 Temporalities and spaces of disability social (in)security

Australia and the UK compared

Chris Grover and Karen Soldatic

Neoliberal social (in)securities: placing disability

In this chapter we focus upon developments in social security policy for disabled people in Australia and the UK with the intensification of neoliberalism as policy hegemony in both countries. Our focus is primarily (but not exclusively) upon income replacement benefits – Disability Support Pension (DSP) in Australia and Employment and Support Allowance (ESA) in the UK – for working age disabled people. In line with other authors within this volume, such as Claire Edwards (see Chapter 2), we conceptualise spaces of social (in)security as spaces of social regulation where disabled bodies are regulated to establish, maintain and reproduce social normative relations of power. Thus, our analysis is focused within the space of social security relations and the techniques of governance drawn upon by neoliberal nation states to make and remake impaired bodies into a range of categories that will either grant or deny them access to disability benefits. Additionally, as a comparative analysis, we focus upon the nuanced and differentiated practices that have emerged at the local scale to regulate impaired bodies in response to broader global neoliberal political economic concerns (cf. Harvey 2005).

Penna and O'Brien (2008) argue that neoliberalism has been conceptualised in various ways, including as a discourse, an ideology and a practice. In terms of its relationship to disability neoliberalism is all of these things. It has, for example, harnessed discourses of disgust and abjection to delegitimise disabled people's claims for social security benefits (see Grover and Piggott 2013; Soldatic and Meekosha 2012a; Soldatic and Pini 2009). It has advanced an ideology around the restructuring of capitalist labour markets that are now increasingly precarious and contingent, and which have undermined the disability rights movement struggles for equality and participation within labour markets (Soldatic and Meekosha 2012b). Finally, with the aim of moving disabled people into paid work, it has been used to implement practices that reorder social hierarchies of the impaired body via new technologies of the governance of worklessness (Grover and Soldatic 2012).

This re-ordering of bodies via social security classification regimes articulates neoliberalism's conceptualisation of the relationship between the state and the individual. In this context, neoliberalism is primarily concerned with the freedom of the individual from the coercion of the state through ensuring that the state's role is limited to only those functions that the market is unable to provide, for instance, the production of public goods, law and order, and the provision of minimal welfare benefits and services (see Turner 2008). For neoliberals, societies are most harmonious when individuals are free from the coercion of the state and when, therefore, individuals are able to operate as independent and self-sufficient citizens who take responsibility for their own actions. Indeed, for many neoliberals individuals can only act responsibly when they are free from state intervention (cf. Murray 1990, 1994). Paid work is central to these considerations, for not only is it held to contribute to the principles (such as competition) of market-based activity, it is also held to be the most appropriate means through which individuals can express their responsibility as citizens. Hence, Clarke (2004: 90) observes neoliberalism is committed 'to "putting people to work": expanding the range and variety of labour power that can be used in the continuing expansion of capitalist production and accumulation'.

It is this conjunction of responsibility and the commodification of labour power that has been driving changes to social security regimes for disabled people in both Australia and the UK. In fact, in neoliberal times, nation states, particularly within the Anglo-sphere, have actively sought to redefine who is disabled (Grover and Soldatic 2012). The primary purpose of this process is to restrict the numbers of people who can be *legitimately* positioned outside of paid employment via the disability category. As Roulstone and Morgan have argued in this volume (see Chapter 4), the discursive positioning of some disabled people as being 'truly disabled' and others as 'shirkers and scroungers' (Garthwaite 2012) has created political consent for the retrenchment of disability benefits (Piggott and Grover 2009). In both Australia and the UK this is clearly seen when reference is made to focusing the most 'generous' benefits upon the 'severely disabled' in Australia (Packham 2013) and those people who 'have a severe limitation' in the UK (Department for Work and Pensions [DWP] 2009: 8).

Understanding changes to social security regimes through the lens of neoliberalism, however, has the danger of suggesting either explicitly or implicitly that the changes are similar in Australia and the UK. At the level of the *direction* of change this may be the case. In both nation states more disabled people face greater coercion to make increased efforts to (re-)enter paid employment (Grover and Piggott 2010; Soldatic and Pini 2012). *How* this is, or should, be done though, differs between the two countries. In many senses, these observations reflect the suggestion that while the economic and social transformations congruent with the rise of neoliberal globalisation has involved broader macro-structural regularities (Harvey 2005; Jessop 2002), more sensitive empirical accounts reveal localised practices in implementing the intent of neoliberal governance (Peck 2001; Savage 2000).

The in-depth empirical comparative work of Peck (2001), for instance, provides a rich geographical account of neoliberal social security restructuring that identifies local discourses, ideologies and practices and the effects on poor, working-class subjects on which they are targeted. Mapping the divergent changes to social security benefits across three Anglophone countries (Canada, the UK and the United States), Peck (2001) demonstrates the ways in which neoliberal 'welfare-to-work' practices negotiate local spatial histories and relations, and are transformed in response to these local contingencies. Recent comparative work (for example, Wacquant 2008) have revealed similar processes of local scale differentiation, even with the onset of global pressures to reform nation state social security regimes. These accounts of neoliberal restructuring are exemplary in illustrating the local particularisms of neoliberal governance, where local interpretations, institutions and practices shape and are reshaped by broader socio-relations of power.

Consistent with these arguments, our conceptual framing of disability social security regimes seeks to illustrate particular practices and differentiation of two national regimes, marking out their distinct differences despite the convergence of the underlying rationality of large-scale neoliberal disability restructuring. In doing this, we focus upon the temporal elements of disability social security regimes occurring at the national scale in Australia and the UK. As Jessop (2008) contends, while the spatial turn has enabled an enriched and nuanced analysis of local practices, too often, this has come at the expense of critically distilling the temporal framing of these local, and particular, practices. Czarniawska and Sevón (1996: 21) suggest that 'in every instance when we accentuate space or time, the other aspect is still present, although hidden'. Hence, May and Thrift's (2001: 1) critique of the 'dualism in the foundational categories of Space and Time' and their observation that 'space and time are inextricably linked' (2001: 2). Consistent with such arguments our analysis seeks to illustrate the embedding of temporality into disability social security regimes in two nations that are at the frontier of neoliberal restructuring (Soldatic 2013).

Temporal insecurities: time as complexity and methodology

Recently, Paterson (2012) argued that disability studies has little considered the role of time in shaping the social experience of disability. Drawing upon the work of Adam (2004), he attempts to illustrate the complexity of times that operate in the social world that are experienced differently by disabled people with varying impairments. Paterson's general conclusions are similarly mooted by Soldatic (2013) in her work which maps out the numerous temporalities that operate in the restructuring of disability benefits in Australia. Both of these authors seek to critically draw upon emerging work in the sociologies of time to explore the multiplicity of times, beyond clock time, that are embedded within varying disability spatial relations and which shape, frame and make disabled subjectivities.

Hegemonic conceptualisations of time are that it is a 'decontextualised, asituational abstract exchange value that allows work to be translated into money' under capitalist social relations, and that it is a key mechanism in reinforcing social relations of power (Adam 2004: 38–39). Time, therefore, as a methodological framework is able to reveal the substantive grounding of complex temporalities in neoliberal social security regimes (Jessop 2008). There is not a single time, but a multiplicity of times that disabled people are forced to negotiate, synchronise and choreograph to maintain access to nation state disability social security benefits (Soldatic 2013).

These observations of time are important because nation state social security regimes are *the* administrative spaces that enact state power to classify and categorise diverse bodies into hierarchical relations of power. Social security regimes are unique spaces for governing power as they operate to reflect normative judgements on 'deservedness' (Applebaum 2001), inscribing bodies with variants of economic value (Grover and Piggott 2013; Soldatic and Meekosha 2012b). This ontological aspect of social security regimes 'exists only through and in concrete … in specific times and places' (Jessop 2008: 184). Therefore, any temporal analysis requires grounding within the particular, the concrete and the local. Hence, our comparative analysis is grounded within the spatial particularisms of two nation state social security regimes which have both been framed by the 'neoliberal turn', but which have drawn upon a diverse set of technologies to bring about the similar effects (Grover and Soldatic 2012).

Within these two spatialities we focus upon temporalities by drawing upon time as a governance mechanism under neoliberal reform, albeit administered differentially in the two locales. To do this we must understand the concept of time. Hassan (2010) argues that the 'temporal turn' in the social sciences and humanities can be dated to at least the early 1990s, since which a theoretically rich literature has emerged that seeks to understand time and its economic and social importance. As many have observed (see, for example, Adam 2004; Glennie and Thrift 1996; Jessop 2008; May and Thrift 2001), time is a complex phenomenon. As we shall see, the disciplinary potential of time – that which is often dependent upon the linear measurement of duration through the clock (Hassan 2010) – remains dominant (Jessop 2008; Soldatic 2013). However, it is also the case that the 'multiplicity of time and their patterns of synchronization, continuity and discontinuity and disruption, and … their seemingly competing rhythmic articulations … result in [the] reshaping of the experience of everyday life' (Soldatic 2013: 2).

For disabled people in both Australia and the UK these are pertinent observations. In the neoliberal restructuring of income replacement benefits for such people various temporalities are used to sort the 'truly' disabled from those who in previous years and under previous social security regimes would have been considered disabled enough to be legitimately exempted from labour market participation. However, due to the neoliberalisation of disability benefits disabled people are increasingly defined as unemployed labour, rather than 'disabled'. In this context, there are at least three ways of understanding time that are relevant to social security regimes for disabled people.

First, chronological time is 'a linear time, defined by a succession of instants' (Ricoeur 1980: 171). Within the disability studies arena chronological time has primarily been related in a rather uncritical way to the idea of the life course, and the importance of disability as a category of policy and as a social experience of it (see Heller *et al.* 2012; Priestley 2003 as examples). These accounts assume a 'strict sequence and timing of life's transitions' (Elchardus and Smits

2006: 303), even though within the disability literature it is well recognised that impairment is differentially framed, particularly when issues such as its onset are accounted for. Moreover, Elchardus and Smits (2006: 303) contend that the 'standardised life course as a natural phenomenon ... are normatively anchored, man-made phenomenon, that imposes regularity on life's events and decisions'. Notions of the life course as a standardised 'natural' phenomenon do not recognise that this temporality is shaped by historical periods. The 'life course' and the 'breaking of the body' into key periodisations is not a consistent historical phenomenon. It is socially constructed and reconstructed, shaped by broader macrostructures of power. Nation state social security regimes reinforce this normative framing around political economic concerns that are historically embedded. It is difficult to find, for example, a clearer exposition of this than recent Organisation for Economic Co-operation and Development (OECD) efforts to extend the retirement age for workers arguing that it is necessary to sustain social security funds (OECD 2012), an argument and practice in the UK that preceded the OECD's publication by several years (for example, Secretary of State for Work and Pensions 2006a).

A second notion of time is 'waiting time'. Waiting time has dominated medical research, particularly in regards to the hospitalisation of patients; that is, the flow through of bodies 'into the system to receive a set of necessary medical procedures "in time" to assure lifesaving treatment' (Savage and Wright 2003: 332). Interestingly, within disability sociologies, there has been little attention paid to the role of 'waiting time' as a neoliberal governing technology in social security regimes. This is a curious omission of the disability research, given, for example, that there have been media reports from the UK that a number of disabled people have died while waiting to be (re)assessed for income replacement disability benefits (Black Triangle Campaign 2012).

The limited attention paid to the relationship between the waiting time for benefits (assessment for, and access to, payments and so on) and disability relations of power within neoliberal restructuring is arguably associated with the normative expectations that frame waiting time. Adam (1990: 121) argues that the dominant tendency to naturalise our experience of waiting time is typically framed around knowing that things can take time due to the processes that they entail. In other words, these processes are often culturally and socially ritualised, such as waiting for the bus, waiting for the mail to come and so on. These ritualised practices of 'waiting time', however, are reliant upon knowledge about processes they entail. They contain in other words a set of expectations. However, waiting time, as we have seen via media coverage and disability activism around social security regimes, is not value neutral and underpinned by an agreed period of time. Thus, the question becomes, 'who waits for whom and how does waiting reflect the broader asymmetrical social relations of power whereby the process of waiting is a ritualised practice to reinforce disciplinary action?' (Schwartz 1974: 842–3). These questions are broadly reflective of Thompson's (1967) original thesis on time, where it is positioned as a mechanism to discipline bodies within capitalist economies and societies.

This leads to a third temporal framing; the relationship between the disability category and work time. Writers, such as Stone (1984), have eloquently captured the ways in which the disability category was initially devised to separate those who could work under the emerging capitalist economy and those people deemed as being unable to compete under these conditions. Work time was shaped and defined by the temporal demands of the political economy, where work was structured around both the speed of the factory and the length of time spent at and in work (Thompson 1967). As Marx (1990: 401) once contended, the speed of labour processes not only had an effect on the body, but also enacted to establish new and emergent social divisions of labour. That is, which bodies were included within the new industrial political economy and which were to remain outside as they were unable to maintain their bodily velocity in time with production and which, therefore, were to be confined to the practices and institutions of the poor law.

While appeals to work time may appear as an outdated mode of analysis, as Jessop (2008) has suggested, new temporal structures have emerged under neoliberal structures of capital mobility and governance. Making a profit in neoliberal capitalism – from the just-in-time production of contemporary manufacturing to the rhythms of the service sector – are as beset by work time as early manufacturing was. In this sense, proving disability to receive income replacement benefits involves 'a test of temporal competency, predictability and sychronicity' (Soldatic 2013: 4) in the context of neoliberal labour markets that, because they are held to be denoted by 'flexibility', are thought to be more conducive to the employment of disabled people.

In the following sections we focus upon what appears to be one – the temporal aspects of disability social (in)security spaces – of the primary points of difference in state re-regulation of disabled bodies through neoliberal intensification. Our analysis empirically delineates the ways in which neoliberal states harness a range of temporalities to govern disabled people. Further, the analysis suggests that while this may be a general trend, temporal technologies of governance are not homogenous, but are locally differentiated and particular. When comparing Australian and UK disability social security regimes, chronological age, waiting time and work time appear to dominant both landscapes as a technology of neoliberal governance, but they remain locally distinct. Finally, what the analysis suggests is that disabled people are required to synchronise the rhythms of their bodies, navigate a range of spatial complexities, and subordinate their familial and community commitments to these three different times.

Time, age and entitlements

There can be little doubt that chronological time, in particular that related to the life course, is central to welfare states and societies. While, for example, there have been many changes to the UK's welfare state since the 1940s, it is still possible, albeit in a rather selective and often diluted way, to view some remnants of Beveridge's (1942) idea of state-organised benefits and services 'from the cradle to the grave'. In this sense, therefore, chronological time has been particularly important in defining those temporalities in which 'dependency' (either upon parents in the case of children and the state/family or market in the case of retirement) has been seen as legitimate, and when (usually referred to as 'working age' – from the school leaving age to the age at which the state retirement pension becomes payable) 'dependency' on anything other than wage work is deemed problematic.

In both Australia and the UK disabled children are provided for through financial support directed towards their parents. This is the case for both income replacement benefits (where parents are not in work or are in poorly paid work) and 'additional cost' benefits to help relieve the extra financial costs that being disabled brings. The way in which the payment of such benefits is calculated is also related to chronological time, although in this instance, it is related to the amount of time spent caring. The 'additional cost' benefit in Australia (Carer Allowance), for example, is paid on the basis of 'time spent on caring' for children which means that not all carers will be eligible for the benefit, despite the time they may spend on caring for someone with the same disability type, as they do not report meeting the time spent of care minimum threshold. While some disability types are listed as potentially eligible for parents (thus, it is assumed that they require the same level of parental care), parents still need to demonstrate the time spent on caring and meet the temporal threshold. In the claim process for Disability Living Allowance for children in the UK comparisons are made to the amount of time an 'average' child may need care for and reference is made to temporal measures (for example, 'continual', 'frequent' and 'prolonged') of the care requirements of disabled children compared to the 'average' and are related to the time (during the day or night or both) that children require caring for.

In Australia the chronological age of 16 as a marker to determine Carer Allowance is also the qualifying age for disabled people to access the Disability Support Pension (DSP) in their own right. The DSP payment system, however, is stratified into a range of categories premised upon different temporal demarcations. The process entails a payment increase with chronological age which ranges from 16–18 years, 18–20 years and 21 years above and these are further stratified into place of residence (within the parental home or living independently). Disabled parents under 21 years receive the same payment level as those 21 years and above. Moreover, payment indexation increases are tied to the age categorisation; under 21 years of age without children rises annually, while post-21 years is indexed twice yearly, resulting in a growing discrepancy between the different age categories. These age-tiered payment rates have existed since the introduction of the DSP in the early 1990s. However, the tiered indexation rates are new.

In the UK social assistance has similar age markers, although its inflationary increase structure is simpler; everyone gets the same (low) rate of increase (currently held at 1 per cent per annum). However, Employment Support Allowance (ESA) does not have categories linked so closely to chronological time. It was argued when first announced that ESA would be paid at a lower rate for younger people (to reduce potential incentives to move between benefits as young people – under the age of 25 years – are generally paid lower rates of out-of-work benefits). This suggestion, though, was heavily criticised for being 'a direct attack on a group of people who are among the poorest in our society, impoverishing them still further' (evidence from the Down's Syndrome Society to the Secretary of State for Work and Pensions (2006b: 15)). The then government suggested that it was not its intention to 'penalise young people' so the idea was dropped (Secretary of State for Work and Pensions 2006b: 20). While in keeping with the general principle of the development of ESA (that there should not be financial incentives for people to move between benefits for unemployed and disabled people), however, a reduced level was introduced for the under 25s that was set at the same level as that for unemployed youngsters for the first three months (what is known as the 'assessment phase') of an ESA claim. After that they are paid at the same rate as older people in the same circumstances.

In Australia the age of 35 is important because in July 2012, the Gillard Labor government 'fast tracked' new workfirst activity requirements for existing DSP recipients under 35 years (Macklin and Australian Government Canberra 2010). DSP claimants under 35 years are now required to meet a strict set of conditions and attend regular compulsory interviews to maintain access to the DSP (Macklin and Australian Government Canberra 2010). For those seeking entry onto the DSP under 35 years, a more stringent entry criteria was introduced, requiring this category of disabled people to wait up to 36 months prior to gaining access to the DSP (Whiteford 2011). This category of disabled people are referred automatically onto the lower unemployment benefit – NewStart Allowance (PWD Australia 2011) – which contains a range of compulsory requirements, such as attending regular interviews. Access to the DSP for this group of disabled people is now conditional on successive failure to find a job. Only those 'so severely disabled' under 35 years automatically qualify in the first instance.

In the UK there has not been an attempt to specifically restrict income replacement benefits for the under 35s (beyond that noted above), although there are restrictions for the under 35s in other benefits (for instance, benefits to help to pay for rent in the private sector). However, the Welfare Reform Act 2012 did detrimentally affect young ESA recipients when special rules allowing young disabled people (aged 16–19 and, in exceptional circumstances, up to the age of 25) to access the contributory version of ESA, even if they had not paid enough national insurance contributions to receive it, were abolished. This concession – what was known as the 'youth provision' – was essentially a continuation of concerns from the 1970s that some disabled people (including those people disabled from birth or childhood) would never access social insurance benefits if they had not been in a position to pay national insurance contributions. For Burchardt (1999: 14), the 'youth provision' is 'best understood as an earnings-replacement benefit, although it may be the lack of potential to earn or engage in other productive activity that is being compensated, rather than the loss of any actual earnings'.

The UK government's own figures suggest that the abolition of the youth provision will result in a loss of income for 80 per cent of people benefiting from it (DWP 2011). For the majority (87.5 per cent) this will be a part loss of income. For others (12.5 per cent), it will mean a loss of the whole of their income. Beyond these recent changes and, unlike the case of Australia, there is no additional wait-ing time for young people claiming income replacement benefits on the grounds of disability.

Qualifying for benefits: time in and at work, and social security access

Australia has had one of the longest running disability pension schemes among Anglophone countries (Grover and Soldatic 2012). The original scheme, based upon a medical assessment of bodily incapacity was, as we have seen, radically transformed in the early 1990s, along with the large-scale restructuring of the Australian social security system (Soldatic 2010). The advent of changes was stimulated by a strong interest in curtailing further growth in the numbers of peo-ple accessing the scheme (Clear 2000). The new social security regime for dis-abled people – the DSP – instituted a combined disability test, entailing a medical impairment assessment, alongside a capacity to work test. Embedded within it was a temporal work test.

The new temporally dependent work capacity test positioned the criteria that established work capacity against full-time work, defined as the equivalent of 30 hours of labour market participation. As Clear and Gleeson (2001) rightly con-tend, the then Labor government's intention was to make the DSP harder to access in order to divert more disabled people into the labour market. It would do this by reducing the number of people accessing, and increasing the number of people leaving, it. In brief, the changes were aimed at making disabled people conform as much as possible to work time. Despite these efforts, by the early 2000s, the numbers on the DSP had grown by over 300,000 in less than ten years (Yeend 2011). The conservative Howard Liberal–National Coalition government once again targeted the DSP for radical reform, and passed through parliament changes to the temporal element of the work test, meaning that people only had to be deemed capable of working 15 hours per week, rather than 30 hours, to be denied it (Soldatic and Chapman 2010).

The effects were significant. The leading Australian welfare agency, ACOSS, for instance, estimate that in 2007–8, a third (35 per cent) of DSP applications were rejected because of this change (ACOSS 2012). However, despite the sig-nificant numbers being deemed 'ineligible' for the DSP, the Gillard Labor gov-ernment announced further changes, with an estimated saving of $624 million over forward estimates (ACOSS 2012). This substantial saving was to come from denying, as we have noted, young disabled people under the age of 35 DSP for the first 36 months of disability if they are deemed capable of working at least eight hours per week (PWD Australia 2011).

In some senses, the UK's Work Capability Assessment (WCA) is less struc-tured by such temporal issues than the Australian system. The focus of the WCA is upon the ability of the applicant to do any work, rather than being able to work for a certain number of hours per week. Despite the fact that part-time work has become increasingly common in recent years in the UK and there is currently concern about under-employment (the enforced working of part-time hours), the WCA does not attempt to denote whether disabled people are capable of working full-time or part-time. They are determined by the WCA to either be capable of working (and therefore, have to claim the UK's unemployment-related benefit, Jobseeker's Allowance, or find paid employment) or they are adjudged not to be capable of paid work, but capable of engaging in mandatory activities to help them secure paid work, or to 'have a severe limitation which creates a significant disability in relation to the labour market, regardless of any adaptation they may make or support with which they may be provided' (DWP 2009: 8). In the case of the latter they are deemed to be so disabled that they are exempted from making efforts that might increase their opportunity to do paid work.

The WCA may not relate deemed capability to work to temporal considerations in the UK. However, it is nevertheless the case that it has been possible for many years for people receiving income replacement disability benefits to engage in some paid work. Currently 'permitted work' rules allow people claiming ESA to legitimately work, primarily up to 16 hours per week. There is an (uneasy) balance here between wanting to only pay ESA to those people 'genuinely' unable to work, but also allowing such people to 'undertake, or try, some work whilst continuing to receive benefits but with … an emphasis on helping them to progress to full-time employment over time' (Dewson *et al.* 2005: 1).

Conclusion: time, space and the neoliberalisation of disability welfare regimes

This chapter has explored a range of times and how the social security regimes of Australia and the UK, as spaces for (re-)regulating disabled people, are, at least in part, structured through temporal concerns related to various notions of time. These observations raise a number of issues related to spatialised temporalities, and the ordering and remaking of impaired bodies to enable access to disability social security benefits. In particular, they highlight the varying temporalities at play and the ways in which these coincide as complex technologies of governance to normatively shape social expectations around access to disability social security benefits.

First, the observations suggest that what are often presented as being discreet 'typologies' of time are not as discreet as might be presupposed. Where, for example, the boundaries of chronological, waiting and work time lie is difficult to analyse, for the same concrete time might represent several of these notions of time and may be influenced by all of them. So, for example, while the age-dependent structures of benefit receipt may be understood as being related to chronological time (in particular in relation to the transition between phases in the life course), they might equally be understood as being 'waiting time'; people awaiting the transition from one part of the life course to another and, in some instances, most notable in Australia's differential treatment of over and under 35 year olds, from one set of entitlement rules (unable to work eight hours per week to unable to work 15 hours per week). Similarly, in the case of the UK, the lower payment for young disabled benefit claimants compared to those over the age of 25 in the first three months of an ESA claim is as much structured through waiting to establish entitlement to ESA (and not providing any incentive to move from the UK's unemployment-related benefit to ESA) as it is concerned with chronological time as its age-related basis might suggest.

Moreover, both chronological and waiting time are overlaid by concerns with work time. Work time, as we have seen, helps to constitute the rhythms of labour markets. The majority of the changes that we have discussed in this chapter have been driven by labour discipline concerns with enforcing work time. While in both Australia and the UK developments in income replacement benefits for disabled people have been justified through paternalistic arguments (they are good for disabled people) and even social justice-type arguments (they will help to reduce inequalities between disabled and non-disabled people), their primary aim has been to ensure that only those people who can be 'truly' understood as disabled, as measured by functional impairment to do paid work, are included in the disability category. The rest, the vast majority, in both Australia and the UK are expected to work or to make efforts to do so.

While concerns with the constitution and enforcement of work time are not new to social security regimes for disabled people (see, for example, Borsay's [2005] account of relief disabled people in workhouses), the imperatives of neoliberalism have demanded a redefinition of the disability category. This has involved a restatement of traditional liberal concerns with the freedom and responsibilities of individuals to support themselves and, if they have one, their families through their own effort, primarily in paid work. In Australia, for example, governments of the left and right have made work central to disability inclusion directives and even access to the new support scheme is premised upon work activation of some kind (Productivity Commission 2011), while in the UK recent governments of different political varieties have also made it clear that financial support for disabled people must activate 'responsible' behaviour, particularly towards paid work (Secretary of State for Work and Pensions 2006b, 2008). Through demanding personal responsibility, not only it is thought by policy-makers that the alleged moral malaise facing the UK (what Conservative ministers refer to as 'broken Britain') will be addressed, but it will help to keep in check the financial costs (and, therefore, the coerciveness of direct taxation) of supporting disabled people. All this is done through the commodification of the labour power of disabled people, which, as we have seen at a general level, is central to neoliberalism (Clarke 2004).

The aim in both Australia and the UK, therefore, is to make the rhythm of disabled bodies, their 'temporal competency, predictability and synchronicity' as we have seen Soldatic (2013: 4) describes it, more in time with those of neoliberal labour markets. The problem is that for many disabled people these two rhythms are not particularly compatible. In various ways, the work capability assessments that govern access to income replacement benefits for disabled people reflect this through their temporal concerns with the 'normal' body. So, for example, in the UK the handbook for health care professionals (HCPs) conducting the WCA is replete with reference to considering the rhythms of disabled bodies with regard to 'reasonable' timescales related to the rhythms of 'normal' bodies (DWP 2012). However, given the large proportions of people now being denied income replacement benefits in the UK, it is clear that many HCPs do not adjudge the rhythms of disabled bodies to be that different to non-disabled people and, therefore, that different to the requirements of neoliberal labour markets. The issue then becomes one of employer perception of whether the rhythm of disabled people's bodies fits with the needs of their enterprises so that disabled people are not considered potentially problematic employees.

Second, it is clear from our discussion that while neoliberalism has a global logic, it is experienced and practised differently in different countries. In Australia and the UK, for instance, changes to the social security regimes for disabled people have been driven by the neoliberal emphasis upon the market and the private. Hence, the general direction of policy travel has been similar in the two countries. As we have noted, the danger with such an approach that emphasises the global nature and logic of neoliberalism as a discourse and a set of practices is that the homogeneity of the embodiment of neoliberalism in particular national states is overplayed (Harvey 2005). Indeed, in many senses, the idea of the global promotion and impact of neoliberalism and the freedom of movement of capital within it, is to suggest that nations, particularly national governments, are to some extent redundant in their functions. So, for example, Jessop (1994a, 1994b) points to the 'hollowing out' potential of changes in the spatiality of economic regulation in late modern times through the usurping of the role of the nation state by supra-national and intra-national forms of regulation and governance. However, as Jessop (1994a, 1994b) and others (for example, Clarke 2004; Harvey 2005) note, it is also the case that the ways in which neoliberalism becomes embodied at a national level is framed by cultural, historical, political and social considerations that are particular to nation states. Hence, the way in which neoliberalism is practised will vary significantly between nations (Peck 2001). These national particularisms around neoliberal state restructuring point to Clarke's (2004: 95–96) observations that 'neo-liberalism has to negotiate other political formations, other political legacies and the political forces and blocs in which they have been embedded'.

The implications of these observations are that, on the one hand, similarities between nations in the development of social security policies might be expected. This is especially so, given in our case that, while its nature is often difficult to discern, there has nonetheless been policy transfer between Australia and the UK (for discussion see Grover and Soldatic 2012; Peck and Theodore 2001; Pierson 2003). We see a convergence in Australia and the UK at a discursive level through the construction of workless disabled people via discourses of social disgust (Grover and Piggott 2013; Soldatic and Meekosha 2012b; Soldatic and Pini 2009) and at the level of practice through what we have seen are moves to a more restrictive disability category. On the other hand, we might expect to see differences in policy as policy-makers struggle with similar dilemmas, framed by the pressures of neoliberalism, within two nation states that have different cultural, institutional and political histories. Hence, while it is the case that there are similarities in the trend of policies for workless disabled people in Australia and the UK at a macro level, there are differences at a micro level (i.e. in the detail of policy).

In our particular case we have focused upon those differences related to temporal structures within social security regimes for disabled people. We have seen that while overlaid with ensuring as many disabled people as possible partake in work time, or at least take part in activities to increase their potential to compete to partake in work time, there are different temporal rhythms to the Australian and UK approaches. In Australia, for example, income replacement benefits for disabled people are more structured through concerns with the amount of time that disabled people might be expected to work for each week, while in the UK the focus is more upon whether disabled people can be considered to be capable of doing any work at all. Furthermore, we have seen differences in the ways in which chronological time is employed differently for disabled people, with, for example, people under the age of 35 being expected to fulfil different qualifying criteria to those over the age of 35. Such age-dependent differences specifically for disabled people are less obvious in the UK's system.

The differences between the two systems reflect the complex material, moral, political and social bases of social security provision in the two countries. We have seen, for example, that an attempt in the UK to pay a lower rate of ESA to the under 25s was deemed politically not possible because of accusations that the poorest young disabled people would be hit particularly hard by the change. Later, and constructed through austerity-related discourses (for example, appeals to 'fairness' and a need for simplification in the social security system (DWP 2011)) young people were adversely affected by the abolition of the youth provision for the contributory version of the ESA. This demonstrates the importance of time to the political process; of waiting for the opportune moment to introduce what are known for claimants to be problematic policies.

References

Adam, B 1990, *Time and social theory*, Polity Press, Cambridge.

Adam, B 2004, *Time*, Polity Press, Cambridge.

Applebaum, L 2001, 'The influence of perceived deservingness on policy decisions regarding aid to the poor', *Political Psychology*, vol. 22, no. 3, pp. 419–442.

Australian Council of Social Services (ACOSS) 2012, *OECD joins growing call for increase in Newstart allowance*, press release, accessed 17 December 2012, www.acoss. org.au/media/release/oecd_joins_growing_call_for_increase_in_newstart_allowance.

Beveridge, W 1942, *Social insurance and allied services*, Cmd. 6404, HMSO, London.

Black Triangle Campaign 2012, accessed 14 March 2012, http://blacktrianglecampaign.org.

Borsay, A 2005, *Disability and social policy in Britain since 1750*, Palgrave Macmillan, Basingstoke.

Burchardt, T 1999, *The evolution of disability benefits in the UK: re-weighting the basket*, CASEpaper CASE 26, Centre for Analysis of Social Exclusion, London School of Economics, London.

Clarke, J 2004, *Changing welfare, changing states: new directions in social policy*, Sage, London.

Clear, M 2000, *Promises, promises: disability and the terms of inclusion*, Federation Press, Sydney.

Clear, M and Gleeson, B 2001, 'Disability and materialist embodiment', *Journal of Australian Political Economy*, vol. 49, no. 1, pp. 34–55.

Czarniawska, B and Sevón, G 1996, *Translating organizational change*, De Gruyter, Berlin.

Dewson, S, Davis, S and Loukas, G 2005, *Final outcomes from the Permitted Work Rules*, Research Report No 268, Corporate Document Services, Leeds.

Department for Work and Pensions (DWP) 2009, *Work capability assessment internal review report of the working group commissioned by the Department for Work and Pensions*, DWP, London.

Department for Work and Pensions (DWP) 2011, *Employment and Support Allowance (ESA) 'youth' National Insurance qualification condition. Equality impact assessment*, DWP, London.

Department for Work and Pensions (DWP) 2012, *Revised WCA Handbook ESA (Amendment regulations) 2011 and 2012*, DWP, London.

Elchardus, M and Smits, W 2006, 'The persistence of the standardized life cycle', *Time Society*, vol. 15, no. 303, pp. 303–326.

Garthwaite, K 2012, 'The language of shirkers and scroungers? Talking about illness, disability and Coalition welfare reform', *Disability and Society*, vol. 26, no. 3, pp. 369–372.

Glennie, P and Thrift, N 1996, 'Reworking E. P. Thompson's time, work-discipline and industrial capitalism', *Time and Society*, vol. 5, no. 3, pp. 275–299.

Grover, C and Piggott, L 2010, 'From Incapacity Benefit to Employment and Support Allowance: social sorting, sick and impaired people and social security', *Policy Studies* (special edition, *Fit for Work? Challenges for the Welfare Reform Agenda*), vol. 31, no. 2, pp. 265–282.

Grover, C and Piggott, L 2013, 'Disability and social (in)security: emotions, contradictions of "inclusion" and Employment and Support Allowance', *Social Policy and Society*, vol. 12, no. 3, pp. 369–380.

Grover, C and Soldatic, K 2012, 'Neoliberal restructuring, disabled people and social (in)security in Australia and Britain', *Scandinavian Journal of Disability Research*, vol. 15, no, 3, pp. 216–232.

Harvey, D 2005, *A brief history of neoliberalism*, Oxford University Press, Oxford.

Hassan, R 2010, 'Globalization and the "temporal turn": recent trends and issues in time studies', *The Korean Journal of Policy Studies*, vol. 25, no. 2, pp. 83–102.

Heller, T, Parker-Harris, S and Albrecht, G 2012, *Disability through the life course*, Sage, Thousand Oaks.

Jessop, B 1994a, 'The transition to post-Fordism and the Schumpeterian workfare state', in R Burrows and B Loader (eds), *Towards a post-Fordist welfare state*, Routledge, London.

Jessop, B 1994b, 'Post-Fordism and the state', in A Amin (ed.), *Post Fordism: a reader*, Blackwell, Oxford.

Jessop, B 2002, *The future of the capitalist state*, Polity Press, Cambridge.

Jessop, B 2008, *State power: a strategic-relational approach*, Polity Press, Cambridge.

Macklin, J and Australian Government Canberra 2010, *Pensions to increase from Monday*, media release, accessed 25 September, http://jennymacklin.fahcsia.gov.au/node/932.

Marx, K 1990, *Capital, volume I* [1867], Penguin Books, London.

May, J and Thrift, N 2001, 'Introduction', in J May and N Thrift (eds), *Timespace: geographies of temporality*, Routledge, London, pp. 1–46.

Murray, C 1990, *The emerging British underclass*, Institute of Economic Affairs Health and Welfare Unit, London.

Murray, C 1994, *Underclass: the crisis deepens*, Institute of Economic Affairs Health and Welfare Unit, London.

Organisation for Economic Co-operation and Development (OECD) 2012, 'Activating jobseekers: how Australia does it', accessed 17 December 2012, www.oecd-ilibrary.org/docserver/download/8113041ec008.pdf?expires =1355728750&id=id&accname=ocid1 77499&checksum=E8CA24200063E9CAC2C43888000F5840.

Packham, B 2013, 'Julia Gillard sheds tears while introducing national disability insurance scheme bill', *The Australian Newspaper*, 15 May, accessed 19 May 2013, www.smh.com.au/business/federal-budget/budget-aftermath-wrap-may-15-2013-20130515-2jlcx.html.

Paterson, K 2012, 'It's about time! Understanding the experience of speech impairment', in N Watson, A Roulstone and C Thomas (eds), *Routledge handbook of disability studies*, Routledge, London, pp. 125–143.

Peck, J 2001, *Workfare states*, Guildford Press, New York.

Peck, J and Theodore, N 2001, 'Exporting workfare/importing welfare-to-work: exploring the politics of Third Way policy transfer', *Political Geography*, vol. 20, pp. 427–460.

Penna, S and O'Brien, M 2008, 'Neoliberalism', in M Gray and S Webb (eds), *Thinking about social work: theories and methods for practice*, Sage, London.

Pierson, C 2003, 'Learning from Labor? Welfare policy transfer between Australia and Britain', *Commonwealth and Comparative Politics*, vol 41, no. 1, pp. 77–100.

Piggott, L and Grover, C 2009, 'Retrenching Incapacity Benefit: Employment Support Allowance and paid work', *Social Policy and Society*, vol. 8, no. 2, pp. 1–12.

Priestley, M 2003, *Disability: a life course approach*, Polity Press, Cambridge.

Productivity Commission 2011, *Disability care and support: inquiry report, no. 54*, Australian Government, Melbourne, pp. 531–561.

PWD Australia 2011, *PWD E-Bulleting*, issue 71, 7 August, People with Disabilities Australia, Strawberry Hills.

Ricoeur, P 1980, 'Narrative time', *Critical Inquiry*, vol. 7, no. 1, pp. 169–190.

Savage, M 2000, *Class analysis and social transformation*, Open University Press, Buckingham.

Savage, E and Wright, D J 2003, 'Moral hazard and adverse selection in Australian private hospitals: 1989–1990', *Journal of Health Economics*, vol. 22, no. 3, pp. 331–359.

Schwartz, B 1974, 'Waiting, exchange and power: the distribution of time in social systems', *American Journal of Sociology*, vol. 79, no. 4, pp. 841–870.

Secretary of State for Work and Pensions 2006a, *Security in retirement: towards a new pensions system*, Cm 6841, The Stationery Office, London.

Secretary of State for Work and Pensions 2006b, *A new deal for welfare: empowering people to work. Consultation report*, Cm 6859, The Stationery Office, London.

Secretary of State for Work and Pensions 2008, *Raising expectations and increasing support: reforming welfare for the future*, Cm 7506, The Stationery Office, London.

Soldatic, K 2010, 'Disability and the Australian neoliberal workfare state', PhD thesis, University of Western Australia, Western Australia.

Soldatic, K 2013, 'Appointment time: disability and neoliberal temporal rationalities', *Critical Sociology*, vol. 39, no. 3, pp. 405–419.

Soldatic K and Chapman A 2010, 'Surviving the assault? The Australian disability movement and the neoliberal workfare state', *Social Movement Studies* (special issue on Australian social movements), vol. 9, no. 2, pp. 136–154.

Soldatic, K and Meekosha, H 2012a, 'Disability and neoliberal state formations', in N Watson, C Thomas and A Roulstone (eds), *Routledge handbook of disability studies*, Routledge, London, pp. 195–210.

Soldatic, K and Meekosha, H 2012b, 'The place of disgust: disability, class and gender in spaces of workfare', *Societies*, vol. 2, no. 3, pp. 139–156.

Soldatic, K and Pini, B 2009, 'The three Ds of welfare reform: disability, disgust and deservingness', *Australian Journal of Human Rights*, vol. 15, no. 1, pp. 76–94.

Soldatic, K and Pini. B 2012, 'Continuity or change? disability policy and the Rudd government', *Social Policy & Society*, vol. 11, no. 2, pp. 183–196.

Stone, D 1984, *The disabled state*, Temple University Press, Philadelphia.

Thompson, E P 1967, 'Time, work-discipline and industrial capitalism', *Past and Present*, vol. 38, no. 1, pp. 56–97.

Turner, R 2008, *Neo-liberal ideology: history, concepts and policies*, Edinburgh University Press, Edinburgh.

Wacquant, L 2008, *Urban outcasts: a comparative sociology of advanced marginality*, Polity Press, Cambridge.

Whiteford, P 2011, 'Will the government slow the growth of disability support pension numbers?', *Inside Story*, 12 May, accessed 20 August 2012, http://inside.org.au/growth-of-disability-support-pension-numbers/.

Yeend, P 2011, 'Budget 2011–12: disability support pension reforms', *Budget Review 2011–12*, accessed 17 December 2012, www.aph.gov.au/About_Parliament/Parliamentary_Departments/Parliamentary_Library/pubs/rp/BudgetReview201112/Disability.

Part II

Experiencing disability, experiencing space and place

6 Part of the problem or part of the solution?

How far do 'reasonable adjustments' guarantee 'inclusive access for disabled customers'?

Donna Reeve

Introduction

Geographers have long recognised that geographies of exclusion are about more than physical exclusion; it is necessary also to consider the role of social, cultural and political discourses in creating and contributing to that (often) unquestioned exclusion (Imrie and Edwards, 2007). In a review of the development of the academic sub-discipline of 'geographies of disability' Imrie and Edwards draw attention to the importance of the relationship between identity and space:

> These types of geographical research point to the recursive relationship between identity and space, by documenting the different ways in which *place is influential in how disabled people feel (about themselves).*
>
> (Imrie and Edwards, 2007: 626, my emphasis)

The concept of 'reasonable adjustments' has been at the centre of UK anti-discrimination legislation designed to give disabled people access to goods and services as laid down by part 3 of the Equality Act 2010 (previously Disability Discrimination Act 1995/2005). This chapter will focus on the ways in which the experience of using reasonable adjustments has an impact on how disabled people feel about themselves because of the messages being provided by the kind of adjustments made. This is done by adopting an understanding of disability (Thomas, 2007: 73) which recognises the impact of disabling barriers which operate at the personal psycho-emotional level (psycho-emotional disablism) in addition to the more usual public structural barriers (structural disablism). Drawing on empirical data I will show how poorly designed and implemented reasonable adjustments can contribute to the level of psycho-emotional disablism in the lives of disabled people. This is particularly evident when considering the provision of accessible toilets which can contribute to the 'indignification' (Imrie and Edwards, 2007: 626) of disabled people. Consequently if a reasonable adjustment is too distressing to use, then the disabled person stays at home – the service provider has simply replaced a structural barrier with a psycho-emotional barrier to inclusion. Examples of 'unreasonable' reasonable adjustments reveal the extent to which disabled people often find themselves in paradoxical landscapes; it *appears* that the built environment is being made accessible as evidenced by numerous signs bearing the wheelchair logo, but disabled people often do not experience the *reality* of this public space as somewhere where they belong (Titchkosky, 2011). So whilst the Equality Act requires that disabled people (and other protected groups) are given access to services in a dignified and respectful manner, it will be suggested that service providers are lagging far behind in their awareness of what this means in practice.

The concept of 'reasonable adjustments' in policy and law

Part 3 of the Disability Discrimination Act 1995 placed duties on service providers that were introduced in three phases. Initially disabled people in the UK had the right to use services and access goods and in 2002 this was extended so that service providers had to make 'reasonable adjustments' for disabled people such as changing the way a service was provided. However it was only in 2004 that the Disability Discrimination Act was extended to impose a duty on service providers to make reasonable adjustments to *physical feature*s which made it difficult for disabled people to access their services (DRC, 2005). For example this has led to the installation of lifts, ramps and loop systems as well as the provision of information in alternative formats for people with visual impairments (although far less often for people with learning difficulties). But it is the term 'reasonable adjustments' which has been at the centre of controversies about the kind of adjustments service providers make, if they make them at all.

It has been argued that building regulations and the Equality Act 2010 (which replaced the Disability Discrimination Act) fail disabled people because there are too many get-out clauses and exemptions. Hence building practices continue to treat accessible design as an 'add-on' or compensatory design (Imrie, 2004) rather than importing inclusive, universal and mainstreaming design precepts into the construction of public space. It is important that these reasonable adjustments restore disabled people's self-esteem, dignity and independence. However in practice it tends to be the last aspect, that of physical access aiding independence, which is concentrated on. Thus the adjustments made are often far from ideal for the people who have to use them.

Roulstone and Prideaux (2009) provide a detailed discussion of the problems caused by the term 'reasonable adjustments' in UK law, policy and practice. There are no 'rule books' about how to make buildings, goods and services accessible to a wide range of disabled people. Consequently the implementations are often subject to the constraints of cost and feasibility rather than with the primary aim of inclusivity.

> Indeed, the use of the provisos 'reasonable', 'practical' and 'impractical' throughout the majority of UK legislation serves to dilute the true extent of the requirements laid down by the DDA [Disability Discrimination Act].
>
> (Roulstone and Prideaux, 2009: 365)

The term '*reasonable* adjustments' was deliberately used within the legislation to ensure that adjustments made to ensure the inclusion of disabled people would evolve over time.

> Service providers should keep the duty and the ways they are meeting the duty under regular review in light of their experience with disabled people wishing to access their services. In this respect it is an evolving duty, and not something that needs simply to be considered once only, and then forgotten. What was originally a reasonable step to take might no longer be sufficient, and the provision of further or different adjustments might then have to be considered.
>
> (EHRC, 2011: 96)

So whilst the term 'reasonable adjustments' is inherently slippery, the intention was to produce an Equality Act which would keep pace with the changing expectations of diverse groups in society. However the term 'reasonable' has been critiqued by disabled people because it facilitates piecemeal 'good enough' adjustments to be made rather than fully inclusive and equal access for disabled people in the spirit of international human rights legislation (Roulstone and Prideaux, 2009). Finally, service providers have to make these adjustments in an anticipatory manner rather than simply responding to the needs of individual disabled people over time. For example, a library that installs text-to-speech software on all their computers enables this public facility to be fully accessible to all people, with and without visual impairments (EHRC, 2011).

However, when thinking about accessibility and reasonable adjustments, the iconic symbol of disability, that of the wheelchair logo, means that typically it is the needs of people with physical impairments who are most likely to be imagined as the 'kind' of disabled people that need to be catered for. Therefore businesses and institutions are much less clued up about the kinds of environmental adjustments that might be needed by people with sensory impairments, learning difficulties, mental health difficulties and social impairments such as autism (Mental Health Network, 2012). Even when these adjustments are made, there is no guarantee of inclusion if the equipment is broken or if the service provider does not know how to use it properly.

Another difficulty is that posed by the conflicting access requirements of people with different impairments. For example blister paving helps people with visual impairments navigate the edges of road crossings but overuse of this tactile paving can make the surface unstable for those with mobility impairments (Department for Transport, 2011). There is no simple answer to this problem and the solution will inevitably be some kind of compromise. However engaging with local groups of disabled people who can provide feedback on the different options available is much more likely to produce reasonable adjustments which are largely acceptable to future disabled customers (EHRC, 2011).

Imrie (2003) highlights the way that architects fail to take account of the physical reality of bodies, the fleshy differences that make up society. If one looks at the plans for urban regeneration, then if people do appear on the prints, they tend to appear in blob form and are intended to give a sense of scale only. Rather than this abstract architectural practice, Imrie suggests that:

> A reflexive architecture is required which is 'open-minded', without bound-aries or borders, and sensitised to the corporealities of the body. An important component of this is for architects to identify the multiplicity of corporeal or postural schemata of the body.
>
> (Imrie, 2003: 64)

I would also add that a reflexive architecture needs to consider the *emotional* impact of using the space being designed; this point will now be developed using the concept of indirect psycho-emotional disablism and returned to frequently in the rest of this chapter.

Indirect psycho-emotional disablism

Historically, disability studies has paid most attention to the experience of struc-tural barriers – documenting the many ways that people with impairments have been prevented from participating and living in mainstream society. This work has deep roots in social policy and sociology and it has been suggested that disability studies has largely neglected *geographical* perspectives on disability (Imrie and Edwards, 2007). Within the sub-discipline of geographies of disability, sophisti-cated understandings have been developed of the complex ways that space, dis-ability and society are interconnected. Writers such as Kitchin (1998) have shown the ways in which inaccessible environments are about more than physical exclu-sion, but also convey powerful messages about being and belonging.

> The ideological messages to disabled people that are inscribed in space through the use of segregationist planning and inaccessible environments is clear – 'you are out of place', 'you are different'. As a result, forms of oppression and their reproduction within ideologies leads to distinct spatiali-ties within the creation of landscapes of exclusion, the boundaries of which are reinforced through a combination of the popularising of cultural represen-tations and the creation of myths.
>
> (Kitchin, 1998: 351)

The experience of moving within 'landscapes of exclusion' is therefore not just about the physicality of the inaccessible built environment, but also produces an emotional effect by reminding someone that they are 'out of place'. So when considering the experience of disabling environments, it is about what is seen, touched and experienced emotionally (Smith, 1999).

This interconnection between the physicality of disabling environments and their impact on the emotional well-being of a disabled person has also been developed within disability studies. Thomas (2007) has developed a definition of disablism which includes reference to disabling barriers operating at the psycho-emotional level (psycho-emotional disablism) alongside the more usual structural/material barriers (structural disablism) associated with the 'traditional' social model of disability.

> The oppression that disabled people experience operates on the 'inside' as well as on the 'outside': it is about being made to feel of lesser value, worthless, unattractive, or disgusting as well it is about 'outside' matters such as being turned down for a job because one is 'disabled', not being able to get one's wheelchair into a shop or onto a bus because of steps, or not being offered the chance of a mainstream education because one has 'special needs'.
>
> (Thomas, 2004: 38–39)

Rather than leaving the experiences of humiliation, shame and anger as emotional problems to be dealt with by psychologists and doctors, these processes of disablement are brought back into the domain of the social; consequently the solutions are to be sought at the level of society/culture rather than down to the individual to manage through therapy.

Psycho-emotional disablism can be broken down into two types – direct and indirect psycho-emotional disablism (Reeve, 2008). The most important form of psycho-emotional disablism is *direct psycho-emotional disablism* which emerges from the interactions that disabled people have with others, such as family, friends, professionals and strangers. Therefore the experience of being stared at for looking 'different', thoughtless comments and invalidating actions can all cause direct psycho-emotional disablism. In addition this form of psycho-emotional disablism includes internalised oppression which can be considered to arise from the relationship that a disabled person has with themselves; the internalisation of the negative messages about disability that are found in the cultural lexicon can lead someone to feel that they are a burden, useless and a second-class citizen.

However for the purposes of this chapter, I want to concentrate on what I have called *indirect psycho-emotional disablism* which arises from the relationship that a disabled person has with the material world. Here, emotional impact arises when disabled people interact with the environment, rather than directly with the shop owner or city architect. Therefore it could be argued that here disabled people are interacting with the *consequences* of the *assumptions* of the shop owner, service provider and city planner – hence the use of the term indirect rather than direct psycho-emotional disablism.

Consequently indirect psycho-emotional disablism would include emotional responses to the experience of disabling structural barriers; the experience of psycho-emotional disablism arises from this reminder that one is 'out of place' because placing someone outside the mainstream in this way can lead to isolation at the psycho-emotional level. Thus this extended social relational definition of disablism devised by Thomas (2007: 73) allows equal recognition to be given here to the structural barriers which prevent someone from *doing* something such as going for a coffee with a friend, as well as the psycho-emotional response to this level of exclusion that prevents someone from *being and belonging* – feelings of anger, hurt, humiliation.

Nonetheless indirect psycho-emotional disablism does not just arise from the direct experience of structural disablism, such as an inaccessible coffee shop. A more insidious form of indirect psycho-emotional disablism can be created when structural barriers are removed and reasonable adjustments are implemented in order to 'include' disabled people. As I will show later in this chapter with some practical examples, the experience of using these reasonable adjustments can be just as disabling as the original structural barriers, continuing to remind the user that they are 'out of place'. Ironically the 'solution' to a physical barrier has created a new psycho-emotional barrier which can maintain social exclusion and isolation if it is too distressing or humiliating to use.

Disabled people are all individuals with their own history and experience. Therefore it should be noted that not all disabled people experience psycho-emotional disablism; it can vary with time and place and is impacted by other aspects of identity such as age, impairment, structural disablism, ethnicity, gender, class and other life events. However as psycho-emotional disablism is akin to emotional abuse (Reeve, 2006), the day-to-day experiences of being reminded that 'you are out of place' can have a detrimental impact on emotional well-being and sense of self. Consequently, psycho-emotional disablism is not simply a 'problem' for the individual to manage, but needs to be acknowledged by academic disciplines and professional groups beyond disability studies/geographies of disability, if disablism at both the public and private level is to be identified and removed.

Indirect psycho-emotional disablism: the reasonableness of 'reasonable adjustments' in practice

I will now look at some of the different ways that reasonable adjustments have been implemented to consider how reasonable these are for the disabled people who use them. Do they facilitate inclusion or serve as another form of exclusion through the creation of indirect psycho-emotional disablism?

Disabled peoples' experience of using 'reasonable adjustments'

Within the remit of the Equality Act (and prior legislation) service providers are required to make reasonable adjustments to their buildings and services so that disabled and non-disabled people have as similar an experience of access, as far as is possible.

> The policy of the Act is not a minimalist policy of simply ensuring that some access is available to disabled people; it is, so far as is reasonably practicable, to approximate the access enjoyed by disabled people to that enjoyed by the rest of the public. The purpose of the duty to make reasonable adjustments is to provide access to a service as close as it is reasonably possible to get to the standard normally offered to the public at large (and their equivalents in relation to associations or the exercise of public functions).
>
> (EHRC, 2011: 90)

It is often assumed that it is very difficult to make historic buildings accessible to disabled people given the need to retain historic context whilst dealing with uneven levels, steps and other physical obstacles. Consequently sometimes the 'solution' to a physical barrier can become rather bizarre as recounted by one wheelchair user who described what happened when he attempted to see an exhibition when he visited Windsor Castle with his family:

> So we went up this ramp, along a narrow corridor, and lo and behold, at the end of the corridor was a lift, only enough for two people. So to get upstairs to have a look around they had to take me out of the wheelchair, dissemble my wheelchair, take the wheelchair up first, sit me on a seat, and then take me up with two guards and my wife, reassemble my wheelchair, and it was the same to come back … So I went to complain and they said, 'You cannot complain, because they've got a lift and they've got a ramp'. It does, it makes you absolutely laugh.
>
> (Robert in Reeve, 2008: 191)

These stories are not uncommon – and whilst this extract could have come from an episode of the 1970s sitcom *Fawlty Towers*, it exposes the ambivalent messages being given to the disabled visitor to this castle. Robert felt disempowered by the fact that the castle had ticked the access box by providing a lift and ramp and so he had no grounds to make a complaint, despite the inconvenience, hassle and physical pain this alternate route to the exhibition caused him. The Equality Act recognises that with respect to physical barriers faced by disabled people, if the physical feature cannot be removed or altered to allow access, then a reasonable adjustment would be to provide an alternative method of providing the service. Therefore when considering Robert's story, it might have made more sense in hindsight to have provided access to the exhibition using audio-visual materials in an accessible room rather than requiring Robert to dismantle his wheelchair to use a lift which was not fit for purpose. English Heritage are an organisation who are the government's statutory adviser on the historic environment in England. Recently they published a guide (Sawyer, 2012) which provides good examples of the creative ways in which historic buildings can be made accessible to diverse groups of disabled people and stresses that commitment to this process has to apply at all levels of the organisation.

Robert also described how redevelopment of his city centre had created a new coffee shop and restaurant which he could only access via a back entrance and staff corridor because no lift had been installed. He found the experience of accessing the coffee shop humiliating to use and some days would decide to stay at home as a consequence.

> And it gets me, you've got all these new premises and they do this and they do that. And you say, 'Are you building a ramp?' 'Oh, it's not on the list'. And that's it then, you just can't get in.
>
> (Robert in Reeve, 2008: 191)

The tendency to implement a tick-box approach to disability access which achieves the bare minimum means that the result will be a building which is not as accessible as it could have been if architects and planners were willing to consider the range of disabled people who might want to purchase food and drink like everyone else. In addition the ticked box makes it difficult for someone such as Robert to challenge the adjustments made on the grounds that they fail to meet the dignity requirement of the Equality Act without involving the law courts and hefty legal bills because of the lack of an officially recognised regulatory body in the UK (Roulstone and Prideaux, 2009).

Unfortunately the 'reasonable adjustments' clause in the law can be used to sanction forms of spatial apartheid which would be unthinkable for any other minority group at the start of the twenty-first century. Whilst the Equality Act is very clear that the duty to provide goods and services to disabled people is an evolving and continuing duty, this is a message which has yet to become fully taken on board by organisations and institutions. In the meantime this spatial apartheid leads to indirect psycho-emotional disablism; negative messages are given to the disabled person about their equal value as a citizen, exacerbated by the lack of legal redress to challenge the service provider.

Finally, other problems occur when disability access *has* been provided, but it is partial and inconsistent. Recent examples of this can be seen in a survey of gym facilities available to disabled people carried out in the aftermath of the 2012 London Paralympics which revealed that disabled people continue to be excluded from access to these facilities (Leonard Cheshire Disability, 2012). So whilst 79 per cent of respondents reported that some kind of accessible parking was available, 31 per cent of respondents reported that counters, tills and tables were inaccessible because they were too high. The consequence of this was that if someone was shorter or used a wheelchair, reception staff were not always aware of their presence and this left them feeling unwelcome and excluded in the sports facility. Lifts are essential to provide access to people with mobility impairments and wheelchair users but only 58 per cent of gyms had audio and tactile facilities in their lift to make it accessible for those with visual impairments. One respondent recounted:

> I once got into a lift and the person I was with told me that beside the controls someone had pinned a photocopy of Braille. Nice to see people are thinking of people with visual impairments but they totally misunderstood how someone would read Braille.
>
> (Respondent in Leonard Cheshire Disability, 2012: 9)

The survey also revealed the importance of staff attitudes and training as to how accessible a sports facility was for disabled customers – if a building is physically accessible, it remains inaccessible if staff fail to meet other access needs such as ensuring that the floor of the gym is kept clear of dumbbells and other equipment which is a trip hazard for people with visual impairments. Not surprisingly it was reported that only 21 per cent of facilities provided information in alternative formats to meet the access needs of people with hearing impairments, visual impairments or learning difficulties.

Disabled people as a separate species? Consequences of the failures of architectural design to include diverse corporealities

In the same way that architectural design needs to be sensitive to the diverse corporealities which make up society (Imrie, 2003), the design of new public buildings in particular needs to be aware of the emotional impact which certain choices can have on members of particular sectors of the community. Unlike older buildings which have to be *modified* to meet the requirements of the Equality Act, the design and implementation of new buildings would be expected to be more inclusive by design, unfettered by existing structural features. In reality, a lack of awareness or concern about responsibilities means this is not always the case. For example, when the design of the National Assembly of Wales' debating chamber was revealed, there was outrage when the design chosen included a flight of steps at the front – this gave a strong message about the implicit link between citizenship and (non-impaired) bodies (Hastings and Thomas, 2005). One local disability activist wrote:

> Mistakes were made in the initial design specification which stated, that 'the building should be open and accessible to the public – including those with disabilities.' 'Including those with disabilities', what are we, a separate species? Do we still not have the right in the year 2006 to be treated as equal citizens of this country, to be fully included as members of the 'public?'.
>
> (Farmer, 2006: 4)

This failure to produce a design for an accessible government building at the start of the twenty-first century, despite legislation, building regulations and government rhetoric about how disabled people are to be fully included members of society by 2025 (Prime Minister's Strategy Unit, 2005), reveals the strength of a 'design apartheid where building form and design are inscribed with the values of an "able-bodied" society' (Imrie, 1998: 129). In the case of the Welsh Assembly building, Hastings and Thomas conclude that:

> professionals and politicians have viewed concerns about access as potential political banana skins, rather than moves in a debate on citizenship. They have done what is felt at any time to be necessary and expedient to ease the passage of an important but potentially troublesome project.
>
> (Hastings and Thomas, 2005: 541–542)

Another disabled woman talked about the debacle surrounding the design of the Welsh Assembly debating chamber and she had a simple message she wanted to send to architects:

> Use your creativity to ensure that there are no steps anywhere, so that everybody gets an easy ride in moving about the built environment. I can't understand that if you have respect for your fellow human beings, that you wouldn't see that.
>
> (Julia in Reeve, 2008: 191)

This lack of respect also upset Robert, what he describes as the 'not doing it', the failing to make simple enabling, rather than psycho-emotionally disabling, adaptations to buildings.

Thankfully organisations are slowly starting to appreciate the significance of both material and psycho-emotional barriers to physical inclusion. One of the new requirements introduced by the Equality Act was that 'public services must treat everyone with dignity and respect' (EHRC, 2011: 14). Consequently when thinking about reasonable adjustments and disabled people:

> The Act requires that any means of avoiding the physical feature must be a 'reasonable' one. Relevant considerations in this respect may include whether the provision of the service in this way significantly offends the *dignity* of disabled people and the extent to which it causes disabled people *inconvenience or anxiety*.
>
> (EHRC, 2011: 106, my emphasis)

The Equality Act aims to provide disabled people with access to services which are as close as possible to those enjoyed by other groups in society. Therefore it is highly questionable whether 'reasonable adjustments' that utilise back entrances to buildings or require a wheelchair to be disassembled in order to use a lift are actually meeting the requirements of the Equality Act. When disabled people are forced to access goods and services in a different manner to other people, it is vital that organisations and institutions consider the emotional impact for the disabled people forced to do this.

Increasingly it is being recognised that reasonable adjustments extend beyond changes to the material world, but also involve education of *people* within the organisation about disability. So for example English Heritage suggest that:

> All staff, and especially those who deal with the public, should be familiar with the requirements of disabled people, and with the facilities available to them. Training of this kind requires a strategic commitment on the part of any organisation and is particularly effective when it is specifically targeted towards each person's role.
>
> (Sawyer, 2012: 46)

If there is an organisation-wide commitment to the value of staff training coupled with the involvement of groups of disabled people as advisors, then it is unlikely that the reasonable adjustments made will replace *structural* barriers with *psycho-emotional* barriers to inclusion.

One of the important advances of the Disability Discrimination Act 2005, which placed a duty on all public bodies to promote disability equality, was that the focus was on change at the *institutional* level rather than on adjustments for *individuals*. Hence public authorities had to think holistically about environments, to plan and evaluate how they were experienced by disabled people and to draw on the expertise of disabled people. Although the Equality Act 2010 has incorporated this duty so that it applies to all groups of people protected under this legislation, the specific duties relating to engagement and analysis of equality impact have since been lost. Therefore the kind of holistic engagement that English Heritage is recommending will be down to the goodwill of the individual service provider rather than being a legal requirement for all to follow.

Accessible toilet provision? The 'indignification' of disabled people

The built environment is not disability neutral but informed by 'spatial practices [that] are characterised by cultural oppression and the indignification of disabled people' (Imrie and Edwards, 2007: 626). Nowhere is this seen more starkly than in the (lack of) provision of accessible public toilets. The rise of modernity led to the requirement for toilets which could be used when outside the home; however the provision of public toilets for social groups such as women and homeless people was relatively late and fragmented, often only instigated as a consequence of civil rights campaigns (Kitchin and Law, 2001). Making the link between public toilet provision and citizenship, Kitchin and Law (2001) argue that in the case of disabled people, this comes down to the separate but related issues of access and dignity. In order to participate fully in society, disabled people, like women and homeless people, need to be able to use toilets which are accessible. However what 'accessible' means in practice can vary with well-documented examples of such toilets being poorly designed, badly maintained, having restricted times of access and being used as storage facilities (Hanson *et al.*, 2007).

Serlin (2010) argues that the 'accessible toilet' erases gender identity for disabled people because it represents a 'type of *non*male space that is conspicuously neither publicly male nor privately female' (Serlin, 2010: 176, emphasis in original). In addition the common provision of accessible toilets in the same physical location as toilets for women – as indicated by the sign 'ladies and disabled toilet' – reinforces the link of dependency by grouping together disabled people and women as separate to men. Given that the issue of public toilets was high on the agenda of disabled activists fighting for social inclusion in the 1970s, Serlin comments that many of these disabled people were:

> surely willing to take on and accept the terms of a deliberately delineated sexual difference if it meant being able to use a public toilet in the first place.
> (Serlin, 2010: 181)

Whilst accepting that this was a pragmatic solution in the 1970s it may be time 40 years later to revisit this tacit acceptance of gender neutral accessible toilets and to instead move towards single-occupancy unisex facilities which would be used by all people – men, women, transgender and disabled people.

Lack of accessible toilets, like any other environmental barrier, results in the exclusion of some disabled people from a full social and work life as movement outside the home has to be restricted to the availability of toilets. A night out with friends might be limited to the one pub in town with a (reliable) accessible toilet.

But in addition to the question of accessibility, there is also the issue of dignity. For example it is not uncommon for accessible toilets in pubs and restaurants to be locked. One pub in my town keeps the accessible toilet locked to prevent people having sex in the extra-large space offered by the accessible toilet and disabled patrons are requested to ask for the key from bar staff. In addition to the embarrassment of having to ask for the key in front of inebriated strangers, the experience is akin to a schoolchild raising their hand in infant school for permission to use the toilet. This is an example of indirect psycho-emotional disablism – having to negotiate access to a locked toilet in this way is humiliating and embarrassing, and people with invisible impairments might also have to argue their entitlement to use this accessible toilet. It also serves to remind users of these facilities of their physical difference because this kind of toilet provision is only experienced by disabled people. Other people at the pub can use the upstairs toilets at a time of their choosing, discreetly, without needing to bring the private act of elimination to the attention of strangers. Kitchin and Law suggest that the way in which disabled toilet provision is legislated for separately reflects the second-class citizenship associated with disability:

> If disabled people were equally valued members of society, then all toilets would be accessible and their provision would not be an issue and would not need to be legislated. Clearly, however, the second-class citizenship bestowed on disabled people is accepted unproblematically by most of the general population.
>
> (Kitchin and Law, 2001: 295)

But it is possible to occasionally reverse the shame; at one conference I attended, there was a single key available to access the corridor to all toilets which meant that it soon became known (rather vocally) as the 'wee key' – a small example of resistance to this form of indignification.

The universal wheelchair symbol: an 'icon of access'?

In the examples discussed above I have shown the ways in which moving within particular spaces, especially those that are created as a response to the legal requirement for 'reasonable adjustments', are often far from reasonable to use. In her book called *The question of access*, Titchkosky (2011) unpacks the blue and white symbol of a wheelchair user which is a universal marker for accessibility. Taking her university as the space to be explored, she notices that these signs for accessibility are often found in places which are inaccessible. For example, a wheelchair sign marks an accessible parking space, but the door near the parking space is too heavy and narrow to use. So whilst the wheelchair symbol is 'like an icon of access' (Titchkosky, 2011: 63), it does not *guarantee* access, merely the *hope* of access. Moreover, the sign serves as a reminder of the continued exclusion of disabled people, 'the normalcy of inaccessibility' (Titchkosky, 2011: 67) – if society were fully wheelchair accessible for example, then the wheelchair symbol would not be needed.

> The icon of access appears, and in so doing it appears as a sign of access made through the social expectation of inaccessibility.
>
> (Titchkosky, 2011: 66)

As I have written elsewhere (Reeve, 2008), the wheelchair symbol also serves to legitimate some forms of bodily difference over others. People with hidden impairments who do not match the stereotypical disabled person who is a wheelchair user and/or older person can find themselves challenged by others when they use facilities such as accessible toilets or disabled parking spaces. Consequently someone may decide to adopt a visible marker of disability such as a stick, or to exaggerate an impairment by 'limping well', in order to use these facilities without harassment – but this can also come with an accompanying emotional cost in publicly identifying as disabled (Reeve, 2002).

I have argued that access to the built environment for many disabled people is partial, a possibility rather than a certainty. When reasonable adjustments are made, they can be humiliating to use, enforcing spatial apartheid and serving as reminders of difference rather than inclusion. As was shown by Robert's comment earlier, it can be difficult to challenge the kinds of adjustments made to make the built environment accessible to disabled people because of the vagaries of the law. So it is not sufficient to pass laws that give disabled people access to the same buildings, goods and services as other people – it is also necessary to provide clear technical access codes and proper enforcement of the law (Roulstone and Prideaux, 2009). Unfortunately, in the UK at least, employers, businesses, town planners and builders (who also need to take account of Part M of the Building Regulations) are left to envisage what is meant by 'reasonable adjustments'; these decisions will be informed at least in part by prejudice and notions of 'who' disabled people are, as well as financial constraints.

There also appears to be a failure to imagine what it would be like to use the 'reasonable adjustments' being made – in the examples I have discussed, whilst access has been provided in principle, the reality of moving within landscapes modified by this add-on style of compensatory design can cause indirect psycho-emotional disablism. The shame and humiliation I experience when having to ask for the key to the toilet at a crowded bar is infantilising and degrading – would the owner of the pub feel comfortable being forced to ask for permission in this way? At the start of the twenty-first century we still have reasonable adjustments to the built environment which lead to forms of spatial apartheid which again serve to remind disabled people of their second-class status in society.

Whilst acknowledging that the new Equality Act specifically includes reference to dignity and respect when defining 'reasonable adjustments', it will take time for service providers to recognise the potential for psycho-emotional disablism in the adjustments they make for disabled people. But until service providers recognise the reality and impact of this hidden form of disablism, disabled people will continue to be faced with reasonable adjustments which reveal at best lack of thought, such as the photocopy of Braille designed to make the lift accessible for people with visual impairments. Finally, in my town there is a pharmacy which has two signs in the front window. There is a blue sign which reads 'Inclusive Access for Disabled Customers', with small icons underneath referring to wheelchair users, people with mobility impairments, hearing and visual impairments. Next to this sign there is a green notice complete with wheelchair logo which says 'please press button for assistance or use the disabled access at the rear of the building' with an arrow showing which way to go. However the button has been broken or vandalised, so that option is not available to the wheelchair user. Therefore the 'inclusive access' means that for some disabled customers in 2013, this equates to 'enter around the back'.

Conclusion

In this chapter I have discussed the difficulties posed by the 'reasonable adjustments' available under law to give disabled people equal access to buildings, goods and services. Spatial politics, accessibility and reasonable adjustments require engagement at an interdisciplinary level and necessitate mixing academia with policy and practice. I have drawn on both disability studies and geographies of disability literature to unpack the origins, development and implementation of 'reasonable adjustments' showing the complexities and contradictions which can result in the built environment. Hence the 'reasonable adjustments' may be far from reasonable to use for the disabled person concerned, illustrating the way in which 'mainstream spaces are often disabling, in emotional as well as material ways' (Chouinard *et al.*, 2010: 4).

Now that the Equality Act has included reference to respect and dignity in the legal definition of what constitutes a 'reasonable adjustment', service providers will be forced to rethink solutions to disability access which are upsetting and humiliating for disabled people to use. Whilst this change in the law is welcomed, it is difficult to see how this extension of 'reasonable adjustments' will be enforced given the history of 'ambivalence exhibited towards planned solutions to equality issues' (Roulstone and Prideaux, 2009: 366).

> Thus, the requirement is for political, policy and legal measures to be strengthened further to ensure that the continuum of interpretations of 'reasonable' is narrowed to reflect the intuitive sense that exclusive environments are increasingly unacceptable.
>
> (Roulstone and Prideaux, 2009: 375)

The failure of service providers to imagine what it would be like to use the reasonable adjustments they implement suggests that it will be a long time before the 'normalcy of inaccessibility' (Titchkosky, 2011: 67) is overturned and disabled people have the same *certainty* of dignity and respect when accessing goods and services as non-disabled people currently have in society. It will be a while before disabled people can rely on 'Inclusive Access for Disabled Customers'.

'Reasonable adjustments' can only achieve full inclusion if account is taken of structural *and* psycho-emotional disablism. Otherwise there is the risk that removing a physical barrier to accessing goods and services is simply replaced with another barrier which operates at the psycho-emotional level – the disabled person remains excluded from full participation. It is also important to acknowledge that indirect psycho-emotional disablism caused by inaccessible buildings or undignified 'accessible' entrances will exacerbate existing direct psycho-emotional disablism in the life of a disabled person. For example Robert already felt like a second-class citizen because of the way that friends avoided him now he was disabled – this negative impact on his self-esteem was reinforced when he was forced to use the back entrance to the coffee shop and restaurant.

Ironically much psycho-emotional disablism is relatively cheap to remove compared to structural barriers because it involves changing minds, not buildings. Therefore it is a form of disablism which every service provider could begin addressing immediately. In many respects the English Heritage guide (Sawyer, 2012) is doing just this by recommending that awareness and education about disability needs to be carried out at every level of an organisation. It is to be hoped that this education of organisations coupled with the involvement of organisations of disabled people as advisors will make the implementation of forms of spatial apartheid increasingly a thing of the past, except as a genuine last resort. Moreover when reasonable adjustments are treated as an ongoing, evolving responsibility for the service provider, then they are less likely to be treated as a one-off tickbox exercise that 'does disability access'. Consequently the adjustments made are more likely to be actually *reasonable* and when managing the access needs of a diverse community, reasonable compromises are more likely to be made that include as many disabled people as possible. Having the right mindset, attitudes and intentions towards genuine, respectful inclusion is paramount.

References

Chouinard, V, Hall, E and Wilton, R 2010, 'Introduction: towards enabling geographies', in V Chouinard, E Hall and R Wilton (eds), *Towards enabling geographies: 'disabled' bodies and minds in society and space*, Ashgate, Farnham, pp. 1–21.

Department for Transport 2011, *Shared space: local transport note 1/11*, The Stationery Office, London.

DRC 2005, 'Ten years of the DDA – November 2005', *Disability Rights Commission*, accessed 25 March 2006, www.drc.gov.uk/emailbulletin/bulletin_42.asp.

EHRC 2011, *Equality Act 2010 statutory code of practice: services, public functions and associations*, Equality and Human Rights Commission, London.

Farmer, Y 2006, 'National Assembly for Wales Senedd building, Cardiff: how compliant is this building?', *Cardiff & Vale Coalition of Disabled People Coalition News*, vol. 2, pp. 3–4.

Hanson, J, Bichard, J A and Greed, C 2007, *The accessible toilet design resource*, University College London (UCL), London.

Hastings, J and Thomas, H 2005, 'Accessing the nation: disability, political inclusion and built form', *Urban Studies*, vol. 42, no. 3, pp. 527–544.

Imrie, R 1998, 'Oppression, disability and access in the built environment', in T Shakespeare (ed.), *The disability reader: social science perspectives*, Cassell, London, pp. 129–146.

Imrie, R 2003, 'Architects' conceptions of the human body', *Environment and Planning D: Society and Space*, vol. 21, no. 1, pp. 47–65.

Imrie, R 2004, 'From universal to inclusive design in the built environment', in J Swain, S French, C Barnes and C Thomas (eds), *Disabling barriers: enabling environments*, 2nd edn, Sage Publications, London, pp. 279–284.

Imrie, R and Edwards, C 2007, 'The geographies of disability: reflections on the development of a sub-discipline', *Geography Compass*, vol. 1, no. 3, pp. 623–640.

Kitchin, R 1998, '"Out of place", "knowing one's place": space, power and the exclusion of disabled people', *Disability and Society*, vol. 13, no. 3, pp. 343–356.

Kitchin, R and Law, R 2001, 'The socio-spatial construction of (in)accessible public toilets', *Urban Studies*, vol. 38, no. 2, pp. 287–298.

Leonard Cheshire Disability 2012, *Does your gym work out for disabled people?*, Leonard Cheshire Disability, London.

Mental Health Network 2012, *Equally accessible? Making mental health services more accessible for learning disabled or autistic people (briefing, issue 255)*, The NHS Confederation, London.

Prime Minister's Strategy Unit 2005, 'Improving the life chances of disabled people', *Prime Minister's Strategy Unit*, 31 July 2006, accessed 16 May 2014, http://webarchive.nationalarchives.gov.uk/+/http://www.cabinetoffice.gov.uk/media/cabinetoffice/strategy/assets/disability.pdf.

Reeve, D 2002, 'Negotiating psycho-emotional dimensions of disability and their influence on identity constructions', *Disability and Society*, vol. 17, no. 5, pp. 493–508.

Reeve, D 2006, 'Towards a psychology of disability: the emotional effects of living in a disabling society', in D Goodley and R Lawthom (eds), *Disability and psychology: critical introductions and reflections*, Palgrave, London, pp. 94–107.

Reeve, D 2008, 'Negotiating disability in everyday life: the experience of psycho-emotional disablism', PhD thesis, Lancaster University, Lancaster.

Roulstone, A and Prideaux, S 2009, 'Constructing reasonableness: environmental access policy for disabled wheelchair users in four European Union countries', *Alter – European Journal of Disability Research*, vol. 3, no. 2, pp. 360–377.

Sawyer, A 2012, *Easy access to historic buildings*, English Heritage, Swindon.

Serlin, D 2010, 'Pissing with pity: disability, gender and the public toilet', in H Molotch and L Norén (eds), *Toilet: public restrooms and the politics of sharing*, New York University Press, New York, pp. 167–185.

Smith, R G 1999, 'Reflections on a journey: geographical perspectives on disability', in M Jones and L A B Marks (eds), *Disability, divers-ability and legal change*, Martinus Nijhoff Publishers, The Hague, pp. 49–64.

Thomas, C 2004, 'Developing the social relational in the social model of disability: a theoretical agenda', in C Barnes and G Mercer (eds), *Implementing the social model of disability: theory and research*, The Disability Press, Leeds, pp. 32–47.

Thomas, C 2007, *Sociologies of disability and illness: contested ideas in disability studies and medical sociology*, Palgrave Macmillan, Basingstoke.

Titchkosky, T 2011, *The question of access: disability, space, meaning*, University of Toronto Press, Toronto.

7 Biographies of place

Challenging official spatial constructions of sickness and disability

Jon Warren and Kayleigh Garthwaite

Background and context

In this chapter we ask a range of related questions. Why do some localities have a much higher incidence of impairment and chronic illness than others? Why do social policy initiatives and health interventions work in some areas and make little impact elsewhere? This chapter will argue that a critical disability studies perspective is required in order to challenge official spatial constructions of sickness and disability. It will confront the way in which public health researchers and geographers have tended to focus on composition or contextual effects (Macintyre *et al.* 2002) instead of seeking a more integrated understanding of spaces and places, as is required when taking a critical disability studies perspective. This chapter will argue that there is a need to understand places as possessing specific identities with intersections between environment, history and culture: a 'biography of place' (Warren 2011). The core of this idea is that places have biographies in the same way as individuals. Furthermore, the intersection of individual and spatial biographies is particularly significant for understanding the structure and impact of disabling barriers. Additionally, relations between collective and individual biographies matter. The relationship between place and the potential individuals have to improve their personal situation and overcome barriers within spaces that have been shaped by a wider collective biography must also be considered. The implications of this approach will be considered by exploring a case study of the former mining district of Easington in County Durham, North East England, UK. In conclusion, we argue that employing the notion of a 'biography of place' has the potential to result in innovative, more effective and better targeted social policy interventions that challenge disabling barriers not only at the level of the individual but also attempt to address barriers which affect entire localities.

Introduction

Within a social model approach to disability, all factors operating beyond the individual merit consideration as all meso- and macro-level phenomena contribute to how an individual is disabled within society. As has been well documented and discussed, the experience of disability is mediated and mitigated by factors such as social class, gender, ethnicity (Barnes *et al.* 1999). However, what has received much less attention from disability studies has been the significance of place as a variable through which the lived experience of disability can be viewed. Geographical analyses of the labour market, health and social deprivation in the UK show us that location is highly significant and that major inequalities are evident. Unsurprisingly then, within a social model analysis it follows that some places are more disabling than others.

Disability is bound up with issues of impairment which are entwined with issues of health and sickness. It is important to point out that whilst these categories interact and overlap, being within one of these groups does not always indicate membership of one of the other categories. For example, individuals may be disabled without having significant health problems; individuals may see themselves as sick but not disabled due to the nature of their health condition. Disabled individuals' impairments may mean that bouts of relatively good health are punctuated by periods of chronic ill health. Alternatively, ill health may in time become chronic conditions which may lead to disability. This fuzzy and often problematic interplay between disability and ill health is further complicated by the administrative arrangements of health and welfare systems. For example, in the UK to be a registered disabled person allows the individuals access to services and bestows certain legal rights against discrimination which those who are 'ill' do not enjoy.

However, what is clear is that disabled people living within communities which are also characterised by poor health are likely to experience additional barriers than if they were living within communities without wider health issues. Consequently, how disability, health and locality interact contribute to the continued construction of biographies of both individuals and places. Personal histories are both constrained and enabled by the character of place. Place, in turn, is shaped by, and actively shapes, the health of residents and visitors (Andrews and Kearns 2005: 2710). Accordingly, we need to search for ways in which histories are etched in the record of places and, cumulatively, contribute to the local 'becoming' of place (Pred 1984). The lesson for those seeking to understand the relationship between individuals and the places they inhabit is that these histories are intertwined with all the processes that contribute to the evolution of a place, and to its character. As a result, environment, history and culture and their intersections are key points for research. Indeed, it is only by understanding the past that it is possible to understand the future. An understanding of a place's past and the processes of how it developed is required if we are to understand its present and the situations of those whose lives are played out within it.

Conventionally, this has been of concern to health geography researchers. Health geographers have tended to focus on composition or contextual effects in an attempt to explain the variations between places (Macintyre *et al.* 2002). Typically, compositional explanations draw attention to the characteristics of individuals concentrated in particular places; compositional factors most frequently examined are indicators of socio-economic status such as individuals' social class, housing tenure, employment status, educational status, marital status, and so on.

Contextual explanations point towards opportunity structures in the local physical and social environment (Macintyre *et al.* 2002: 130). Whilst this allows insights about what may be going on within spaces, these insights are limited as they do not dispute the way in which place is conceptualised. This chapter argues that there is a need to look at the issue in another way to understand places as characterised by specific identities rather than attempting to explain health variations as deviations from a 'normal' or 'standard' place; an assumption which has been central to social policy interventions. Accounting for such differences requires a view of place as something which is constituted by history, geography, industry, culture and the combined interweaving lives of those living within an area. For example Dennis *et al.* (1956) outlined how the coal industry developed ways by which industry recognised and accommodated the negative health impacts upon its workers, moving older men to lighter work and surface duties rather than excluding them from the workplace on grounds of health. In mining and many other heavy industries, ill health was a fact of working life but also actively managed, thus benefitting the community and the industry. Yet once this industry no longer existed, communities were left without their major employer and with a legacy of chronic health problems and no viable strategy for addressing these problems. An approach which actively critiques and takes issue with conventional ideas about disability, health, place and space is required. Such an approach is wholly consistent with a social model approach to disability. In doing so, the concept of a 'biography of place' will be outlined, and its implications for policy explained.

What makes a place?

As a starting point, it is important to consider the basic question: 'What is a place?' Gersmehl (2008: 60) supplies us with a definition in its most basic form, arguing that a place is: 'an area with definite or indefinite boundaries or a portion of space which has a name in an area'. This definition is helpful but not because it provides a detailed definition; instead, it is useful as it illustrates the ambiguous nature of place, highlighting how places are the products of wider social processes and broader political forces; how places are defined and by whom are essential to making sense of them. Official definitions of place essentially see them as containers of population, and these containers have usually been designed to serve a purpose which has been defined externally. For example, UK parliamentary constituencies are based upon the need to contain an optimum number of citizens. Other examples include Local Authority wards or the boundaries of local authorities. Living on the margins of a place may prove highly significant as moving across a boundary may mean an individual is subject to higher taxation or unable to qualify for additional place targeted initiatives (Cummins, J *et al.* 2007).

The above discussion shows how place is constructed; this may be seen as a benign process or, as we wish to argue, indicative of wider hegemonic forces. Place is conceptualised and constructed to be part of the social apparatus which Finkelstein (1993) termed the 'administrative model' of disability. In order to counter this dominant narrative, within which place is essentially a passive category which the state and its agents use in order to commodify individuals and communities as part of broader structures of governmentality, a radical reconceptualisation of place that is consistent with a critical disability studies approach and the social model is needed in order to challenge this hegemony. To do this it is necessary to see place as the canvas upon which the lived experience of disability is written, in order to understand its role in shaping that experience. Disability studies has produced detailed and important critiques of the built environment, housing, transport (see authors such as Dyck 1995; Gleeson 1999; Hall 2000; Imrie 1996; and Smith 1997), and the assumptions inherent within these systems, together with the way disabled people have been excluded from many arenas. It is clear that these insights can be used in order to understand the relationship between space and disability on a broader conceptual level. The place within which sickness and disability is experienced is not just a container; it is something which is highly active and significant in determining the nature of that experience. For those engaged with social policy, this means that place cannot be taken for granted. Place is not a ready-made container within which potential solutions and initiatives can be delivered. Instead, the nature of a place needs to be an essential part of those initiatives and interventions.

Policy landscape

The above discussions must be situated within the vastly changing policy landscape for sick and disabled people across the UK. Although it would not be viable to succinctly summarise the entirety of changes to the UK benefits system here, it is important to briefly note some key facts and figures. In the UK in November 2012, the working age early estimates of sickness benefits recipients was 2.4 million (Department for Work and Pensions [DWP] 2012). The key sickness benefits are: Employment and Support Allowance (ESA) for new claimants from October 2008, and Incapacity Benefit (IB), which provides support for people who cannot work because of an illness or disability which started before October 2008. Under the ESA regime, new claimants must undergo the Work Capability Assessment (WCA) carried out by private company Atos Healthcare. From April 2011, IB recipients have also started to undertake this assessment.

Further reforms were declared in the Welfare Reform Act, which set out a variety of short- and longer-term strategies intended to contribute to spending reductions, including the replacement of Disability Living Allowance (DLA), a non-means-tested, non-contributory benefit available to help with extra costs disabled people can incur, with a more rigorously tested Personal Independence Payment (PIP) in 2013. Eligibility for a range of benefits is being restricted, alongside reductions in the actual levels of specific benefits being paid, whilst strategies have been designed to incentivise individuals to move off benefits where possible. For example, an overall cap has also been introduced, limiting the total amount of benefits that can be claimed to no more than the average earnings of a working family: £500 per week for couples and lone parents and £350 per week for single adults. Among measures designed to make the welfare system more efficient, the introduction of a Universal Credit, from 2013, stands out. This will provide a single streamlined payment for people of working age, aimed at improving work incentives. The government is introducing a range of other changes intended to incentivise employment for those considered capable of work. These proposed changes have significant implications for sick and disabled people given disabled people's greater reliance on out-of-work benefits and housing benefits than non-disabled people. This is significant as welfare reform has been shown to affect certain areas more adversely than others. Beyond the largest cities, County Durham is set to lose nearly £190m a year in benefit income (Beatty and Fothergill 2013: 14), illustrating that the experience of the reforms will impact in varying ways according to place.

Towards a biography of place?

Whilst place is not solely determined by the bureaucratic and administrative needs of the state and its institutions, these pressures are extremely powerful in shaping what it is and in setting the limits of how it can be imagined. Oliver and Barnes (2012: 120), in their discussion of the importance of definitions, quote Hahn (1985: 94) who goes as far to argue that 'fundamentally disability is defined by public policy. In other words, disability is whatever policy says it is'. The above statement is recognisable when considering the way in which place is also often subsumed by the needs of policy-makers, with place becoming 'whatever policy says it is'. Consequently, there is a need to re-imagine place in order to provide a viable counter-narrative to the dominant narrative which sees place as little more than an administrative category which in turn has led to a failure to challenge the 'one policy fits all' approach that national governments have pursued in Britain since the early twentieth century which asserts both the complexity of and the importance of understanding place. In order to begin this process we can usefully draw on what Wright Mills (1959) termed the 'Sociological Imagination', asserting that 'no social study that does not come back to the problems of biography, of history and of their intersections within a society has completed its intellectual journey' (1959: 4). Wright Mills' seminal text was first published over half a century ago but his arguments are just as valid today as they were then, perhaps even more so. Mills also contended that 'neither the life of an individual nor the history of a society can be understood without understanding both' (1959: 5). This statement about how the history of society shapes the lives of individuals is applicable not only to whole societies but to communities, and in order to fully comprehend the health of those who live in a place, we need to understand that place; not only the history but the narratives of work, locality, culture and being. It is these parts which can be said to constitute a 'biography of place'. For example Mills urged us to study the critical points where biography and history intersect and the junctures where private troubles become public issues. Mills made this point with his discussion of unemployment. To understand unemployment in a place such as Easington, which we discuss in depth later in the chapter, space is highly significant as its labour market was dominated by a declining industry within a regional context of industrial decline for most of the twentieth century. Without an account of place the dynamics between personal trouble and public issue would be unintelligible. It is important to point out that this biography is more than just the sum of these parts; neither is it a 'one way street'. Wright Mills also viewed the action of individuals as shaping the social structures they inhabit:

> By the fact of his living he contributes, however minutely to the shaping of society and to the course of its history, even as he is made by society and its historical push and shove.
>
> (Wright Mills 1959: 6)

In order to explain the present in a locality and the lives of those who reside there, it is necessary to understand the area's past as well as the individual and collective past. It is also significant to recognise that the ways in which a place has been conceptualised and administered are part of this process and how this can contribute to the biography of a place. Our argument does not wish to deny this, but it does seek to show that these processes are only part of a wider story which needs to be understood. Biographies of place become embedded over time and are revealed and manifested in individual life stories.

With regard to issues of health, illness and disability the effects of working in particular conditions or the lack of work, experiencing an environment, living in certain types of housing stock are all recognised social determinants of health and well-being (Marmot 2010). This newfound readiness to acknowledge the significance of social factors is encouraging and opens up a potentially fruitful opportunity for a dialogue between disability studies and critical public health. It would appear to be self-evident that the underlying circumstances and characteristics of a place need to be considered before potential solutions are offered; this may be an area where we can learn something from medical practice. For example, medicine routinely takes patient histories in order to diagnose problems and prescribe remedies. Within medicine, it is accepted that whilst there may be an accepted course of treatment for a condition, the way in which it is applied to individuals will vary, according to their present condition, prior experiences and behaviours. We propose that the same process is required for places. When applied to places, such an approach allows a path to be trodden between the 'one size fits all' approach which discounts difference, and a 'complexity' approach which see the problems of each place as being a unique and atomised 'case in itself'. Instead, an intervention which draws upon best practice in the policy field but is equally aware of the biography of the place within which an intervention is to be deployed becomes possible.

The idea that context matters to individual health is in itself nothing new. Plentiful research has focused on the respective contributions of contextual and compositional effects (Diez-Roux 1998; Diez-Roux *et al.* 2000; Duncan *et al.* 1993, 1998). A parallel debate on the theoretical constructs underlying community effects as well as on measurement of these effects is also evident (Birch *et al.* 1998; Diehr *et al.* 1993; Diez-Roux 1998; Diez-Roux *et al.* 2000). The origins of these effects may be due to what are frequently termed compositional attributes – the characteristics of people living in certain types of areas (Diez-Roux 2000; Duncan *et al.* 1996, 1998; Macintyre *et al.* 1993). However, Bernard *et al.* (2007) argue that such a polarised debate regarding this framing of effects constitutes an oversimplification. Cummins *et al.* (2007: 1835) suggest that it is imperative to collapse the false dualism of context and composition 'by recognising that there is a mutually reinforcing and reciprocal relationship between people and place'. Having such a view prompts an analysis of processes and interactions that occur between people and the social and physical resources in their environment. They call for more multi-dimensional research that combines multiple ways of under-standing places, including resident reports, systematic observation and objective measures on the location and spatial accessibility of resources (see for example, Hortulanus 2000; Martinez *et al.* 2002; Stafford *et al.* 2005). Alongside this, the significance of qualitative research must not be underestimated and allows for 'insights into how people relate to places and the resources available to them locally' according to Cummins *et al.* (2007: 1826). For example Warren *et al.* (2013) found that users' engagement with a case management service was limited due to the poor quality of public transport links in the area. This was historic-ally the case and also contributed to a reluctance to travel from potential service users.

The above suggests that what is notably missing from discussions is how dis-ability can factor into notions of place and health. It would be incorrect to say disability has been wholly ignored to date; for example, there has been attention paid to the relationships between disability and place. It has been argued that social and political structures marginalise people with physical impairments and produce built forms which further exacerbate both the disablement and the social exclusion associated with impairment (see authors such as Dyck 1995; Gleeson 1999; Hall 2000; Imrie 1996; and Smith 1997). Thus far the non-feminist geo-graphic literature concerned with disability has paid comparatively little atten-tion to such subjective aspects of coming to embody an ill and disabled self in a particular place (Crooks and Chouinard 2006: 347). Instead, the emphasis has been on understanding disability as the objective outcome of social relations and practices which are somehow 'external' to or separate from the process of com-ing to embody (and contest) illness and disability. This work has provided many important insights into the causes and consequences of disablement, including the role of changing class relations in the segregation of disabled people under indus-trial capitalism (Gleeson 1999), the marginalisation of disabled citizens within urban environments as a result of urban design and planning practices catering to the needs of the able-bodied (Imrie 1996), and the role of discriminatory attitudes and practices in the spatial exclusion of disabled people from urban neighbour-hoods (Dear *et al.* 1997; Wilton 2000). However, as Kitchin (1998: 354) argues: 'there is the need for studies which seek to examine and expose the socio-spatial processes which underlie disablist practices'. Therefore, we argue that incorporat-ing a critical disability studies perspective into the idea of a 'biography of place', in order to construct a holistic account of what it is like to live in a particular area with a particular context, is essential. Otherwise, contextual and compositional arguments, whilst to a degree helpful, can be viewed to be essentially attempting to account for a place's deviation from an idealised imagined norm around which an intervention has been designed. Our starting point is to consider each place as unique and then to look at what it may have in common with other places. Privileging one explanation over another, when thinking about the relationship between health and place, and when adopting a critical disability studies perspective, is highly problematic. Such an approach suggests that there is a single cause or a hierarchy of cause and therefore that adequate explanation requires the identification and isolation of *the* cause(s). For example, ill health related worklessness is often the product of a complex interaction of several factors: the environment, the social, the economic and also individual lifestyles: the compositional, the contextual, and beyond. In other words, we need to pay attention to the elements which make up an area's history and culture – its biography.

Easington: a case study

The mid 1980s witnessed deindustrialisation in the UK on a major scale, and in County Durham what is most often reported is the demise of the coal industry and the industrial action associated with this. One of the most important features of this job loss is that it has been virtually all concentrated in just a dozen or so areas across Britain, including Easington and its surrounding areas in County Durham. In most of these areas, coal mining had been the dominant source of employment for men, so the consequences for local labour markets were always going to be serious (Beatty *et al.* 2007: 5). Easington district covers the area of East Durham which lies in the North East of England. The North East of England is a post-industrial area broadly comparable in terms of deprivation and health to areas such as the Welsh Valleys and other ex-mining areas in Europe and the United States. Easington district is also regularly described as post-industrial but that is not a wholly accurate description; East Durham is better described as a 'post-coal' mining area as its last pit, Easington Colliery, closed in 1993. In many ways, the district is typical of the wider North East of England region. In terms of most key economic and social indicators it is either approximately the same or just below the regional average. For example, in Easington in November 2009, receipt of Jobseeker's Allowance (JSA), the main benefit you can receive when someone is out of work and seeking employment, was in line with the North East average of 5.3 per cent. Similarly, in terms of lone parents receiving out-of-work benefits, the figures show that in Easington lone parents account for 2.5 per cent of the population, only half a percentage point higher than the average for the UK. Yet when we examine ill health related worklessness measured in terms of the amount of people claiming incapacity related benefits (key out-of-work benefits for sick and disabled people) things look radically different. Easington has the second highest rate of ESA and IB claims in the country. At 16.3 per cent, the rate is much higher than the North East average of 9.6 per cent and more than double the national average of 7.0 per cent according to the National Online Manpower Information System (NOMIS) 2009.[1]

Mapping Easington's biography allows the legacy of once being a coal mining community to still be a significant factor that can go some way to explaining its high sickness benefits receipt. Disabled people are most likely to be economically inactive in areas with weak labour markets and most likely to be employed in areas with strong labour markets (Beatty *et al.* 2000). The perception that those receiving IB are individuals with health problems who lost jobs in the industrial upheaval in the 1980s and 1990s and, finding themselves unable to find work, were legitimately diverted onto sickness benefits, is at the heart of Beatty and colleagues' popular thesis. Beatty *et al.* (2000) have argued, for example, that regional differences in employment rates conceal forms of 'hidden unemployment'. This concentration of 'hidden unemployment' in former industrial areas suggests that some regional economies have not fully recovered from the fallout of deindustrialisation, a conclusion also reached by a number of other researchers (see Theodore 2007; Turok and Edge 1999; Webster 2006).

Beatty *et al.* argue that the most plausible explanation is a continuing lack of jobs: in these areas the supply of workers outstrips demand, the gender segmentation in the labour market declines with successive cohorts, and we therefore have competition between genders (Beatty *et al.* 2009). Norman and Bambra (2007) recognise that IB may hide unemployment, yet their estimates using census data on economic activity suggest that 'previous assertions about the relationship between IB and unemployment may have been overzealous' (2007: 333). In addition, in areas such as County Durham, it is no longer accurate to talk about a generation of ex-miners living out their lives on sickness benefits, as they are likely to have reached state pension age. Indeed, as Fothergill comments, a generation of ex-industrial workers made redundant in the 1980s and 1990s will finally reach state pension age. In turn, this group of older workers have been replaced by a younger generation of disadvantaged and marginalised workers with health problems (Fothergill 2010: 5).

Constructing a 'biography of place' for Easington

Cultures take time to become established and do not disappear overnight. Easington Colliery has been closed since 1993, but Easington still remains a mining community in many ways, with the habits and culture of previous generations persisting and with good reason. This notion is essentially what Bourdieu termed 'habitus' – a system of 'dispositions' which are lasting ideas about the world acquired from culture and by perception, thought and action, mediating structure and agency (Bourdieu 1977, 1990).

Mining communities, due to the way in which work was the centre of the villages and by the way in which housing was tied to the pit and social life to the miners' welfare clubs, rapidly developed a particular culture (see Dennis *et al.* 1956). Broader cultural attitudes around gender and work may also persist (Smith *et al.* 2010). Mining was from the mid-nineteenth century onwards an exclusively male occupation. Attitudes about what constitutes legitimate 'men's work' and 'women's work' to some extent persist, and this potentially explains the reluctance of men to take up employment on a part-time basis or within service based industries such as call centres which have appeared in the area over the last decade. Further, trying to promote a message about how 'work is good for your health' (Black 2008) in communities where the reality of going to work for many meant risking their lives on a daily basis, and disabled so many, is highly problematic and very likely to be dismissed. This 'reality' or perception of work as an adversary, although now not experienced first-hand by many, has been passed down through generations. For instance, many miners developed chronic health problems as a direct consequence of work, and many had to give up work before retirement. These everyday realities meant, and arguably still mean, that messages to 'stop smoking, eat healthily, and drink less' need to be considered within a context in which life was historically precarious to say the least. As Ackers (1996: 160) comments:

> Today, they [the miners] only inhabit our world as ghosts from a rapidly receding past, so that the near-death of the industry has freed the historian from the uncomfortable but compelling commitment to the day-to-day battle of the living.

Such messages are about what *might* happen in the future but the future for working miners was perceivably a long way off and, given their occupational health risks, something which might never come. Furthermore, chronic and disabling health conditions, particularly respiratory conditions, were seen as almost inevitable and part of the fabric of life in the community which accommodated rather than challenged such impairments.

Perceptions of a particular place can also influence its biography. For example, research exploring the experience of long-term sickness benefits receipt found that the majority of stakeholders who worked with sick and disabled benefits recipients spoke about the aftermath of the collapse of the coal industry for the North East and its impact upon sickness benefit take-up (Garthwaite *et al.* 2013: 5). Below is an extract from an interview with Michael, an occupational therapist for Condition Management Programme (CMP), an initiative which was provided by the now defunct Pathways to Work initiative aimed to help service users manage long-term health issues more effectively. Michael talked about his experiences of working in Easington:

> It's the culture, the culture and the mindset, how people have been growing up having this industry and the belief that it was always gonna be there and in one fell swoop it was gone and it's interesting cos in some of the outlying districts the smaller pits it hasn't affected them the same as say Easington which solely depended upon those pits. I really don't know the answer cos they've pumped millions into Easington, absolute millions and nothing's changed – in fact, it's probably got worse.
>
> (Michael, occupational therapist, CMP)

The above quotation from Michael highlights the significance of culture and its role for disability and health narratives, thus suggesting how a place's biography can permeate the opinions of those working in a particular area.

How can a biography of place inform policy and practice?

Any successful intervention to improve policy needs a robust and wide evidence base. In order to achieve optimum results, a willingness to explore and understand the biography of a place and adapt the solution accordingly, just as medicine takes account of a patient's specific symptoms and history, is required. Improving health, reducing health inequalities and challenging social disabling barriers have traditionally focused on the deficits and problems of individuals and communities. Understanding communities by their high mortality and morbidity rates, high hospital admissions, high crime rates and high worklessness is only seeing part of the picture. The common response to such problems has been to provide more services, valuing professional intervention as the answer, together with a focus on the failure of individuals and local communities. All too easily communities are seen as problem areas, and people as passive recipients of services, almost surviving as consumers to outmanoeuvre the system. Community spirit and networks dissolve and the poor health remains; therefore, it is important to challenge dominant views and promote alternative visions of place.

In contrast, a holistic approach that understands place as something that also has assets acknowledges and identifies the skills, strengths, capacity and knowledge of individuals and the social capital of communities (Foot and Hopkins 2010; Kretzmann and McKnight 1993). Such an approach is capable of providing a different story of place; a story that can provide a positive picture that values what works well and highlights examples of where health and well-being are thriving. Harnessing community pride and spirit and engaging in solutions that are more sustainable for that community, with the help of outside support where it is needed most, makes good sense. Through acknowledging how individuals and communities are contributing to health outcomes, their role as co-producers of health and well-being, as empowered producers and active participants, is enabled. Engagement becomes meaningful and empowering rather than tokenistic and consultative. Within Easington district the 'Health works' community health project provides an excellent example of community engagement and involvement. Commissioned as part of primary care, the centre offers health services but also provides a space for community activities. The service was based upon consultation with the local community who are also involved in the day-to-day running of the centre. Such an approach has the potential to help communities identify their own assets and work collaboratively to develop them, strengthening control, knowledge, self-esteem and social contacts thus giving skills for life and work. However, it must be remembered that not all communities are equal; many will require a great deal of help and support to identify the resources and skills required in order to address associated health issues and disabling barriers.

Conclusion

Much of current thinking and practice on how to tackle disabling barriers and to provide support to those with long-term health issues is both ahistorical and acontextual. Much is already known about areas such as Easington, and there is certainly no shortage of descriptive data from health and local authorities, government agencies and community organisations. The challenge for researchers is to go beyond description and to attempt to unravel the underlying meaning of such data and the complex interplay of space, place and disability which collude to produce the variations which are so noticeable in a place like Easington.

Existing empirical research has been highly effective in putting 'place' firmly on the agenda for health and investigating how social inequalities in health are created and maintained. However, advancing our understanding of how places relate to disability and health will require moving beyond existing conceptualisations of 'place' within both the institutions that create, deploy and administer policy and empirical research. This development is necessary in order to fully comprehend the complex relational spatial interdependencies which exist between people and places. Recognising that individuals can become embedded in multiple health damaging and health promoting environments, across time and space, and at multiple scales is crucial if we are to further understand the importance of 'place' in the generation of health inequalities and the construction and maintenance of disabling barriers.

As this chapter has shown, there is scope to understand the intersections between social, political, cultural and industrial landscapes through the interweaving of personal and place biographies. These entangled landscapes have become embedded over time to shape and reshape collective and individual memory and experience, and ultimately impact upon health and disability narratives within a complex 'biography of place'.

Note

1 Employment and Support Allowance (ESA) is a UK government state benefit which replaced new claims for Incapacity Benefit (IB) and Income Support (IS) on the basis of incapacity for work for most claimants from October 2008. However, the government announced in 2010 that claimants would all be migrated to ESA between spring 2011 and 2014.

References

Ackers, P 1996, 'Life after death: mining history without a coal industry', *Historical Studies in Industrial Relations*, vol. 1, pp. 159–170.
Andrews, G J and Kearns R A 2005, 'Everyday health histories and the making of place: the case of an English coastal town', *Social Science and Medicine*, vol. 60, pp. 2697–2713.
Barnes, C, Mercer, G and Shakespeare, T 1999, *Exploring disability: a sociological introduction*, Polity Press, Cambridge.

Beatty, C and Fothergill, S 2013, 'Hitting the poorest places hardest: the local and regional impact of welfare reform', Centre for Regional Economic and Social Research, Sheffield Hallam University.

Beatty, C, Fothergill, S and Macmillan, R 2000, 'A theory of employment, unemployment and sickness', *Regional Studies*, vol. 34, no. 7, pp. 617–630.

Beatty, C, Fothergill, S and Powell, R 2007, 'Twenty years on: has the economy of the UK coalfields recovered?', *Environment and Planning A*, vol. 39, pp. 1654–1675.

Beatty, C, Fothergill, S, Houston, D, Powell, R and Sissons, P 2009, *Women on incapacity benefits*, Centre for Regional Economic and Social Research, Sheffield Hallam University.

Bernard, P, Charafeddine, R, Frohlich, K, Daniel, M, Kestens, Y and Potvin, L 2007, 'Health inequalities and place: a theoretical conception of neighbourhood', *Social Science & Medicine*, vol. 65, no. 9, pp. 1839–1852.

Birch, S, Stoddart, G and Beland, F 1998, 'Modelling the community as a determinant of health', *Canadian Journal of Public Health*, vol. 89, pp. 402–405.

Black, C 2008, *Working for a healthier tomorrow*, TSO, London.

Bourdieu, P 1977, *Outline of a theory of practice*, Cambridge University Press, Cambridge.

Bourdieu, P 1990, *The logic of practice*, Polity Press, Cambridge.

Crooks, V A and Chouinard, V 2006, 'An embodied geography of disablement: chronically ill women's struggles for enabling places in spaces of health care and daily life', *Health & Place*, vol. 12, no. 3, pp. 345–352.

Cummins, J, Francis, R. and Coffey, R 2007, *Local solutions or postcode lotteries?*, Office of Public Management, London.

Cummins, S, Curtis, S, Diez-Roux, A V and Macintyre, S 2007, 'Understanding and representing "place" in health research: a relational approach', *Social Science & Medicine*, vol. 65, no. 9, pp. 1825–1838.

Dear, M., Gaber, S, Takahashi, L and Wilton, R 1997, 'Seeing people differently: changing constructs of disability and difference', *Environment and Planning D: Society and Space*, vol. 15, pp. 455–480.

Dennis, N, Henriques, F and Slaughter, C 1956, *Coal is our life: an analysis of a Yorkshire mining community*, Tavistock, London.

Department for Work and Pensions (DWP) 2012, *Welfare reform act*, TSO, London.

Diehr, P, Thomas, K, Cheadle, A, Psaty, B M, Wagner, E and Curry, S 1993, 'Do communities differ in health behaviors?', *Journal of Clinical Epidemiology*, vol. 46, pp. 1141–1149.

Diez-Roux, A 1998, 'Bringing back context into epidemiology: variables and fallacies in multi-level analysis', *American Journal of Public Health*, vol. 88, no. 2, pp. 216–222.

Diez-Roux, A V 2000, 'Multilevel analysis in public health research', *Annual Review of Public Health*, vol. 21, pp. 171–192.

Diez-Roux, A V, Link, B and Northridge, M E 2000, 'A multilevel analysis of income inequality and cardiovascular risk factors', *Social Science and Medicine*, vol. 50, pp. 673–687.

Duncan, C, Jones, K and Moon, G 1993, 'Do places matter? A multi-level analysis of regional variations in health-related behaviour in Britain', *Social Science and Medicine*, vol. 37, pp. 725–733.

Duncan, C, Jones, K and Moon, G 1996, 'Health-related behaviour in context: a multilevel modelling approach', *Social Science and Medicine*, vol. 42, pp. 817–830.

Duncan, C, Jones, K and Moon, G 1998, 'Context, composition and heterogeneity: using multilevel models in health research', *Social Science and Medicine*, vol. 46, pp. 97–117.

Dyck, I 1995, 'Putting chronic illness "in place": women immigrants' accounts of their health care', *Geoforum*, vol. 26, no. 3, pp. 247–260.

Finkelstein, V 1993, 'Disability: a social challenge or an administrative responsibility?', in J Swain, V Finkelstein, S French and M Oliver (eds), *Disabling barriers – enabling environments*, Sage Publications and Open University Press, London, pp. 34–43.

Foot, J and Hopkins, T 2010, *A glass half full: how an asset approach can improve community health and wellbeing*, Improvement and Development Agency 2010, London.

Fothergill, S 2010, 'Welfare-to-work: time for a rethink', *People, Place and Policy Online*, vol. 4, no. 1, pp. 3–5.

Garthwaite, K, Bambra, C and Warren, J 2013, '"The unwilling and the unwell"? Exploring stakeholders' perceptions of working with long term sickness benefits recipients', *Disability and Society*, pp. 1–14.

Gersmehl, P 2008, *Teaching geography*, The Guilford Press, New York.

Gleeson, B 1999, *Geographies of disability*, Routledge, London.

Hahn, H 1985, 'Toward a politics of disability: definitions, disciplines, and policies', *The Social Science Journal*, vol. 22, no. 4, pp. 87–105.

Hall, E 2000, '"Blood, brains, and bones": taking the body seriously in the geography of health and impairment', *Area*, vol. 32, no. 1, pp. 21–29.

Hortulanus, R 2000, 'The development of urban neighbourhoods and the benefits of indication systems', *Social Indicators Research*, vol. 50, pp. 209–224.

Imrie, R 1996, *Disability and the city: international perspectives*, St. Martin's Press, New York.

Kitchin, R 1998, '"Out of place", "knowing one's place": space, power and the exclusion of disabled people', *Disability and Society*, vol. 13, no. 3, pp. 343–356.

Kretzmann, J and McKnight, J 1993, *Building communities from the inside out*, ACTA Publications, Chicago.

Macintyre, S, Ellaway, A and Cummins, S 2002, 'Place effects on health: how can we conceptualise, operationalise and measure them?', *Social Science & Medicine*, vol. 55, pp. 125–139.

Macintyre, S, MacIver, S and Sooman, A 1993, 'Area, class and health: should we be focusing on places or people?', *Journal of Social Policy*, vol. 22, pp. 213–234.

Marmot, M 2010, *Fair society, healthy lives: the Marmot review*, University College, London.

Martinez, M L, Black, M M and Starr, R H 2002, 'Factorial structure of the perceived neighborhood scale (PNS): a test of longitudinal invariance', *Journal of Community Psychology*, vol. 30, pp. 23–43.

National Online Manpower Information System (NOMIS) 2009, *Labour market profile for Easington*, July 2008–June 2009, accessed 16 May 2014, www.nomisweb.co.uk.

Norman, P and Bambra, C 2007, 'Incapacity or unemployment? The utility of an administrative data source as an updatable indicator of population health', *Population, Space and Place*, vol. 13, pp. 333–352.

Oliver, M and Barnes, C 2012, *The new politics of disablement*, Palgrave Macmillan, Tavistock.

Pred, A 1984, 'Place as historically contingent process: structuration and the time-geography of becoming places', *Annals of the Association of American Geographers*, vol. 74, pp. 298–307.

Smith, G 1997, 'Reflections on a journey: geographical perspectives on disability', in L Marks and M Jones (eds), *Disability, diversability and legal change*, Kluwer Law International, The Hague, pp. 49–64.

Smith, K E, Bambra, C and Joyce, K E 2010, '"Striking out": shifting labour markets, welfare to work policy and the renegotiation of gender performances', *Critical Social Policy*, vol. 30, pp. 74–98.

Stafford, M, Cummins, S, Macintyre, S, Ellaway, A and Marmot, M 2005, 'Gender differences in the associations between health and neighbourhood environment', *Social Science& Medicine*, vol. 60, pp. 1681–1692.

Theodore, N 2007, 'New Labour at work: long-term unemployment and the geography of opportunity', *Cambridge Journal of Economics*, vol. 31, no. 6, pp. 927–939.

Turok, I and Edge, N 1999, *The jobs gap in Britain's cities: employment loss and labour market consequence*, Policy Press, Bristol.

Warren, J 2011, 'Living the call centre – global, local, work, life, interfaces', doctoral thesis, Durham University.

Warren, J, Garthwaite, K and Bambra, C 2013, '"It was just nice to be able to talk to somebody": long-term Incapacity Benefit recipients' experiences of a case management intervention', *Journal of Public Health*, vol. 35, no. 4, pp. 518–524.

Webster, D 2006, 'Welfare reform: facing up to the geography of worklessness', *Local Economy*, vol. 21, no. 20, pp. 107–116.

Wilton, R 2000, 'Grounding hierarchies of acceptance: the social construction of disability in NIMBY conflicts', *Urban Geography*, vol. 21, pp. 586–608.

Wright Mills, C 1959, *The sociological imagination*, Oxford University Press, New York.

8 Shaping local ethical spaces of care and caring for people with learning disabilities

Edward Hall

Introduction

In the current era in the UK of heavily constrained public spending, and with popular opinion seemingly set against the maintenance of welfare support, many people with learning disabilities (and others) are losing their social care support and a range of benefit payments as eligibility criteria are tightened (Community Care, 2012a). In these difficult times, individuals with learning disabilities are increasingly looking to their families, friends and supporters, and local voluntary organisations, to fill the expanding care gap (*Guardian*, 2013; Hall, 2011). Whilst this is undoubtedly causing hardships for many, the austerity-driven reconfiguration of care and support for disabled people is also generating possible opportunities for new and progressive forms and spaces of care. Importantly, however, the chapter emphasises for there to be such positive outcomes from the current crisis, the political and policy/practice context has to be right. The chapter argues that the form of devolved governance from the UK to Scotland (and other countries of the UK) and onto local authorities and communities has been generative of a new model and landscape of 'care': care broadly conceptualised, co-produced, holistic, locally-based and centred on an 'ethics of care' based on mutuality and trust (Lawson, 2007). This collective and negotiated provision of care is in stark contrast to the personalised and commodified model of social care dominant in England (and in many other neoliberal welfare states), where individuals are given 'personal budgets' to purchase care in a social care marketplace (Hall, 2011), budgets which are now being severely cut.

The chapter will focus on independent community-based actors in Scotland, known as 'Local Area Co-ordinators' (LACs), who are conceptualising and practising a co-productive and ethical model of care (Bartnik and Chalmers, 2007). LACs facilitate and 'broker' care and support for people with learning disabilities within local areas, working with individuals and families, and drawing on the full range of formal services and informal community organisations, to maintain the existing social networks and spaces of people with learning disabilities, and seek out connections and opportunities. These expanded networks of spaces and relations of care and support within local areas, the chapter concludes, can challenge the everyday discrimination, exclusion and abjection experienced by so many, and strengthen senses of belonging and respect for people with learning disabilities.

The chapter draws on data from a research project commissioned by the Scottish Government's Health and Social Care Directorate and the Scottish Consortium for Learning Disability (SCLD) (a partnership of charities and universities) to examine the introduction of 'Self-Directed Support' in Scotland (Scottish Government, 2010). In-depth interviews were held with a range of senior policy and operational staff and LACs; the commissioned research did not include capturing the experiences of people with learning disabilities, the subject of a forthcoming project. This chapter is part of a small, but significant, body of work on learning disability in social geography (Hall and Kearns, 2001; Metzel and Philo, 2005).

The remainder of the chapter is in two main sections: first, a reflection on how devolution to Scotland and onto local areas has shaped a context within which a 'progressive' form of localism and an ethical model of social care can flourish; second, an examination of the practice of LACs in building a 'local ethics of care' of networks and spaces of care and opportunities for people with learning disabilities. The chapter concludes that co-productive working between people with learning disabilities and LACs can offer real possibilities for belonging and valuing of (learning) disabled people within local communities.

Social care for people with learning disabilities in Scotland

The Scottish government has sought to shape a nationally distinctive programme of social policy since its formation in 1999 (Mooney and Scott, 2012), one characterised by universalism and an emphasis on public sector provision (Scottish Government, 2010). This stands in contrast to a vigorous pursuit of the personalisation of social policy in England, with individualised funding at the core. The number of people using Direct Payments – funding given to individuals and families in lieu of social care they would have received from the local authority – has rapidly increased in England (by 35 per cent in 2011–12; Community Care, 2012b), with 432,349 (53 per cent of those eligible) using a Direct Payment in March 2012. In Scotland, in the same period, there were 5,049 in receipt of Direct Payments (Scottish Government, 2012). The low take-up of individual funding in Scotland has been attributed to several factors: limited demand by individuals, a reluctance within some local authority social work departments to promote personalisation (Manthorpe *et al.*, 2011), and what has been claimed is a broader socio-cultural favouring of publicly provided services, and a dislike of becoming involved in markets of social care (Keating, 2005; Mooney and Scott, 2012). The individualised, rights-based, aspirational, financially-centred, understanding of personalisation promoted by the UK government, in partnership with In Control and the major disability charities (Hatton *et al.*, 2008), has, it seems, little purchase in Scotland.

The chapter argues that devolution has permitted, indeed encouraged, the forging of a new path on social policy and the delivery of a non-commodified, co-productive and ethically-based model of social care in Scotland. The open and largely consensual approach to policy-making in devolved Scotland has led to a different articulation of 'personalisation'. The Scottish government's *Self-directed support: a national strategy* (2010), whilst using some of the language of person-alisation, makes the distinction with England clear:

> Self-directed support is seeing people as the whole person and the whole life, and it's not just focused on social care and direct payments.
>
> (Senior Policy Manager, Health and Social Care Directorate, Scottish Government)

Individual funding is included in the National Strategy, indeed it *has* to be as the right to have a Direct Payment remains UK legislation – but crucially it is not placed centrally; it is seen solely as a 'mechanism' (Scottish Government, 2010: 7) to achieve a broader co-productive and holistic model of Self-Directed Support.

> Self-directed support is an active process rather than a passive thing, so it's something that you do rather than something that you get.
>
> (Director, In Control Scotland)

The National Strategy (Scottish Government, 2010) establishes a model of co-production in the provision of social care, involving individuals, families, social work and other related professionals, alongside local authorities, and local volun-tary organisations; defined in the Strategy as:

> Co-production in Self-Directed Support (SDS) is support that is designed and delivered in equal partnership between people and professionals.
>
> (Scottish Government, 2010: 7)

> The definition of SDS relies on co-production in identifying and agreeing outcomes and support plans. There has been a gradual shift in this direc-tion, and social care policy generally reflects the inappropriateness of seeing people as 'users' of a public service which is delivered, relegating them to a passive role which adds little social value, and provides no opportunity for equal participation in our services. Understanding that people have skills, capabilities, knowledge and experience to contribute unleashes huge poten-tial for co-producing better outcomes across public services. Co-production redefines the relationship between public service professionals and their cli-ents: from dependency to mutuality and reciprocity.
>
> (Scottish Government, 2010: 15)

This is distinctly different to the focus on 'aspirational' budget-holding citizens (Raco, 2009) in the model of personalised social care in England. The National Strategy sets out right from the start that 'choice and control' are important to give to people, but that these choices exist in contexts of co-operative (and, of course, at times, problematic) relationships with family, care professionals and others. Further, the 'redefinition' of the care relationship from 'dependency to mutuality and reciprocity' establishes an approach of an 'ethics of care', an approach, as we shall see in the following section, which is proactively translated into practice by LACs.

The National Strategy is signed by both the Scottish Government Minister for Public Health and the Convention of Scottish Local Authorities (COSLA) Spokesperson for Health and Wellbeing; reflecting both the open and consensual process by which the policy was formulated and the central role local authorities will play in devising the details of social care policy in their areas, and in the delivery of social care to people with learning disabilities (and others) within communities. This is an outcome of the 'Concordat' agreement between the Scottish government and local authorities, reflecting a 'fundamental shift in the relationship', in which the government sets out the 'direction of policy and overarching national outcomes', and local authorities deliver services 'to meet varying local needs and circumstances' (Scottish Government and COSLA, 2007: 7). The National Strategy, therefore, sets out the desired but broadly defined outcomes, seeing its role as establishing 'test sites' where Self-Directed Support is actively put in place (Ridley *et al.*, 2011), and encouraging local support organisations and local 'champions' to 'spread the word' (Scottish Government, 2010: 12–18) and become involved in the co-production of social care provision.

> What we think the growth is going to be is through organisations that are a bit independent of the local authority, either user-led organisations or the many organisations that support people by client group having that capacity to know where to go … At the local level you're gonna need champions. You're gonna need champions in the world of the person [with learning disabilities] who uses their own support, and you're going to need champions within the statutory organisations that help spread the word.
> (Senior Policy Manager, Health and Social Care Directorate, Scottish Government)

These 'champions' include LACs, who, as we shall see in the following section, work with people with learning disabilities (and the local authority and the full range of local organisations) to identify and try to achieve their aspirations, promoting their presence within local communities.

Significantly, the National Strategy, whilst developed in a period of relative financial certainty, was launched in the new era of severely constrained public funding. Whilst local authorities in Scotland, as in England, have been forced to restrict access to social care funding through the tightening of 'eligibility criteria' (increasingly restricted to those in 'severe' and 'critical' need) (Community Care, 2012a), unlike in England this has not caused a huge gap in provision to open up. In England, the direct connection made between personal funding and choice and control is hugely problematic when this funding is cut off for more and more people. The more broadly conceived Self-Directed Support focuses on the process of co-production rather than the mechanism of direct payments, and means that in Scotland, although many people are experiencing changes and/or reductions to their services, there has been no 'cliff-edge' in care provision. As social care funding is significantly reduced in England, the central role of individual budgets is generating a crisis in the neoliberal model of personalisation. In Scotland, in contrast, spaces and opportunities are opening up to fashion innovative forms of support beyond local authority funding. In one local authority, North Lanarkshire, there has been an imaginative response to the unavoidable tightening of eligibility criteria, ensuring that those in need of support, but now ineligible for funding, are still considered.

> We have what we call a 'personalised prioritisation framework' that makes judgements about what is eligible and what need we will meet – but the distinction between that and general eligibility criteria is it doesn't then say, 'if your needs come in at a lower priority, it's nothing to do with us'; we will take responsibility to see if your needs can be met in other ways through a whole rich spectrum of different approaches, whether it be peer support or signposting to other universal approaches or whatever it is.
>
> (Senior Manager, North Lanarkshire Council Supported Employment)

Whilst this is certainly a 'model of good practice', and therefore not evident in every local authority, the above does reflect a more inclusive approach to provision of care and support for people with learning disabilities, which, as funding becomes restricted, will become increasingly important. That is, whilst eligibility criteria are used to identify those in 'critical' and 'severe' need, those who now fall outside these criteria, i.e. those with moderate learning disabilities, remain included within the broad framework of Self-Directed Support, but with the emphasis being on sources of support outside the social care funding regime. LACs, the chapter argues, can be lateral thinking social care innovators on the ground to work with people with learning disabilities to build a package of care and support in these new circumstances.

  Whilst the cuts in funding and services are material, and many people with learning disabilities (and many others) are being significantly affected, in Scotland and across the UK, this does not necessarily mean, I wish to argue, the collapse of provision of care and support. The broadening of social care to include a range of organisations, in particular those in the voluntary sector, could be critiqued as an invocation of the Conservative-led Coalition government's notion of the 'Big Society' (Westwood, 2011), as part of its broader 'localism' agenda (Department for Communities and Local Government, 2011). This apparent devolution of responsibility from central government to local areas, and families and individuals, has been greeted with little enthusiasm. Featherstone *et al.* (2012) neatly sum up the reaction of many: '[localism] is being mobilised as part of an anti-state, anti-public discourse to build support for roll-back neo-liberalisation' (177). However, the example of social care within a devolved Scotland – devolved from Westminster to Edinburgh, and then again through the Concordat agreement to local authorities – suggests that localism can actually be generative of a new approach to social care. Levitas (2012), in an attempt to envisage a more 'progressive' understanding of localism, specifically cites care as one way in which localism can be reclaimed. She argues that what we can term 'austerity localism' understands care as a state-delivered formal service and therefore one that can be packaged and delivered by private or voluntary organisations.

A more 'progressive localism' conceives of care as a broad and diverse set of social relationships within a range of spaces and as such, care that is impossible to neatly define and commodify. Whilst funding cuts are real and significant, they are also generating debate over the meaning and provision of care and innovative practices, such as the example of North Lanarkshire above, potentially recasting care as less about the formal, practical 'carer–cared for' relationship (although this remains important), and more about caring for (in the broadest sense) people and places, in what I will now go on to describe as a 'local ethics of care', with the everyday co-productive and proactive practice of LACs at its core.

A local ethics of care for people with learning disabilities: the role of Local Area Co-ordinators

The devolution of governance in Scotland (and many other countries), with local authorities in partnership with other local organisations taking on further responsibilities for the design and delivery of social care, is generating a set of new and innovative spaces of care and caring, beyond the limiting regime of personalisation. This is happening in spite of or, it could be argued, even in part because of the severe cuts to funding in all local authority areas in Scotland and the wider UK. What is emerging, as the evidence below will show, is a landscape of care that is very different to the neoliberal notion of individually funded and managed care that dominates in England and elsewhere: a landscape constituted of a complex weave of spaces and networks of formal and informal care, serving the increasing number of people with learning disabilities and others many (but by no means all) of who are now deemed ineligible to receive funding for care and support.

As the world of care has expanded beyond formal sites – as day centres and supported homes are closing or access to them is being restricted – into the everyday spaces of community organisations, public space and people's homes, there has been a (necessary) broadening out of the conceptualisation of care, beyond the powerful construction of the 'carer–cared for' dyad. In geography, the study of the relations and practices of care in a range of spaces has (almost inevitably) revealed the complex socio-spatial and emotional nature of 'care' and 'caring' (Conradson, 2011). Tronto (1993) has suggested four facets of an expansive notion of care: immediate 'caregiving', the actual practical and emotional provision of care to an individual or group; 'care receiving', the ways in which those in receipt of care respond, either positively or negatively; and beyond this broader notions of 'caring about', that is, being attentive to the needs of others; and 'taking care of', assuming some responsibility for other's needs. This typology helps us to think beyond care as a formal practical act and to view it instead as a common, everyday and wide-ranging set of connections and relations, that we are *all* involved and implicated in, in some form (for example, childcare and volunteering) (Barnes, 2012).

Hughes *et al.* (2005) adopt a feminist perspective to critique the dominant masculinist notion of 'care as dependency', commonly cited by the disability political movement (Morris, 1997), and refocus attention on 'acts of caring' which encompass a much wider range of practices beyond formal sites and relations. Lawson (2007), a geographer, argues that this 'foregrounding [of] social relationships of mutuality and trust' (3) is a particular and positive form of 'ethics of care'.

This is a particularly important moment for such a new understanding of social care to emerge, as the dominant agenda of individualism, choice and control, and rights and citizenship for disabled people begins to show signs of strain, as fewer people are entitled to funding, and progress towards positions of social inclusion (such as paid employment) has stalled. There is an opportunity to shift the discourse on 'care' from individual rights to funding now and personal provision, to building lives centred on social connections and local spaces (Johnson *et al.*, 2010). As Reinders (2000) argues so eloquently, having rights, choice and control 'may open doors, but they do not open hearts'. Further, Braidotti (2012) pushes us to think less about individual choices and control, and more about sustained relationships, a focus on practical action, and an emphasis on positive processes.

Thinking through the perspective of ethics of care reveals the limitations of 'personalised' care and support for 'independent' living for the achievement of a satisfying and sustainable 'good life' (Hall, 2011). Instead, we should be focusing on the social interdependencies we are all enmeshed in, which of course take place within spatial contexts. Geographers have sought to place an ethics of care within particular (and varied) locations (Massey, 2004), in what has been termed an 'ethics of the local' (Gibson-Graham, 2003). As noted above, as formal care services are severely cut and fewer people with learning disabilities are assessed as eligible to receive funding, other individuals and organisations in local areas will begin to fill the gaps in care (albeit incompletely and unevenly). Whilst there will be undoubted hardships for many, as trusted services are cut, the changes will also possibly mean that individuals (and families) will look beyond individualised care services to local organisations, spaces and networks for assistance, drawing upon and producing an ethics of connection and care in local places; as Gibson-Graham (2003) argues, the local area (and its communities, networks and spaces) can become the 'active subject' of caring.

The chapter now turns to what could be an example of a local ethics of care in action. 'Local Area Co-ordinators' (LACs) were one of the key recommendations of *The same as you?* review of learning disability services in Scotland (Scottish Executive, 2000); significantly, their valued role is noted in the new learning disability strategy, *The keys to life* (Scottish Government, 2013). Local Area Co-ordination was intended to provide a network of locally-based organisers or 'brokers' of care and support services for people with learning disabilities, a crucial role being to access and secure opportunities beyond formal services. *The same as you?* identified the role of the LAC as 'a specialist worker dedicated to working with a small number of people using services in one area [to] help people and their families through the current maze of systems' (Scottish Executive, 2000: 12).

Significantly, Local Area Co-ordination was conceived in a context of cuts to formal social care provision. Developed in Western Australia in the late 1980s to replace withdrawn state-funded care services, Local Area Co-ordinators were intended to engender caring networks and strengthen community capacity in local areas to ensure ongoing support for people with learning disabilities so they could remain in their home areas and not be transferred to distant institutional care sites. The originator of LAC, social care innovator Eddie Bartnik, visited Scotland in 1999 at the invitation of the then Scottish Executive; soon after LAC was included in *The same as you?* (Scottish Executive, 2000), an example of the particular character of decision-making in devolved Scotland: open, rapid and largely consensual. The focus of LACs' work is their building of relationships with people with learning disabilities; in doing this they are connecting into and expanding spaces and networks of 'care' beyond formal care, focused on people, relationships, places and local spaces.

> The co-ordinator's role is on many levels – individual, family, agency, community – and includes many areas – housing, employment, health, education. They will co-ordinate services and provide information, family support and funding to individuals and families.
>
> (Scottish Executive, 2000: 19)

The introduction of LACs was a 'recommendation' and not a directive of *The same as you?* (Scottish Executive, 2000), again reflecting the particular nature of devolved government and localism in Scotland. Since 2000 there has been a gradual, but uneven, growth of LACs, from eight in five local authority areas in 2002 to 86 in 21 (of 32) areas in 2012 (therefore, 11 areas, including Dundee, do not have LACs: these local authorities would argue they have staff in equivalent roles) (Scottish Consortium for Learning Disability, 2012a). Drawing on evidence from three local authority areas (named 'East', 'West' and 'Central') in Scotland where the LAC model is in place, the chapter argues that the proactive and co-productive approach adopted by LACs generates an ethically-informed 'carescape' of supportive and encouraging relationships and spaces.

> We do lots of different things; you don't need to go to this person to do that, to that person to do this. We can generally find an 'in' for most people; if we're not the ideal person to see, let's link you in with the person that can. We can support people through things that maybe they're slightly anxious and apprehensive about. Because we're flexible … LACs are a 'jack of all trades' and they can help you with anything.
>
> (LAC 1, East)

> The different areas we have are information and signposting, pointing them in the right direction. Then there are equality issues, which are about overcoming barriers to participation, dealing with discrimination and human rights. You've got your community development which could be on a one-to-one

basis, to get people involved in local groups or social clubs. Accessing formal services could be linking them with the Job Centre, getting people involved with Citizens Advice, Direct Payments, sorting out benefits, filling in housing applications, getting people into volunteering, getting people into work. Then you've got your future life planning, getting people to think about their future.

(LAC, Central)

LACs employ practical, instrumental and, crucially, emotional skills in an attempt to 'help people through the maze' of welfare benefits and social care support, and beyond to their aspirations for independent living, community involvement and, in some cases, employment. This help is provided, however, in a way that reflects the way in which 'care' and care relationships are being reimagined by LACs. Bartnik (along with Ron Chalmers) laid out the 'principles' of Local Area Co-ordination (Bartnik and Chalmers, 2007: 26): the first and most important is to 'build and maintain effective working relationships with individuals, families and communities'. Bartnik and Chalmers used the term 'co-production' (now common in education, for example) to describe the way in which LACs work alongside individuals and families with a shared commitment to action, and a focus on an individual's 'gifts and capacities' rather than their deficits (Hunter and Ritchie, 2007: 17); the LACs interviewed had clearly adopted this principle:

We work with people at their own pace. We go out, meet with somebody, find out where they're at, what's going on in their lives now, and what it is they want to achieve, what's their goal, what's their aspirations for the future, and *then we work out how we would work with that person* to achieve those goals and aspirations. Ask the families and carers as well.

(LAC 1, West; emphasis added)

You might be working with an individual, but you're working with the family unit as well. So, it might be you've got a young person or adult with a [learning] disability and then you start working with them, then you find out mum's got issues, so mum needs help and then you can find out that a brother or sister has issues as well, so you end up working with the whole family unit.

(LAC 1, West)

And to work with that individual you often have to work with the whole picture, because whatever is happening elsewhere is impacting on that person you're working with.

(LAC 2, West)

The above quotes illustrate how LACs work with individuals in three important contexts: first, family and friendship, and carer and supporter networks, which are a central feature of the everyday lives of people with learning disabilities (Power, 2008); second, the local place and spaces within which the individual lives and the continued valuing, for some, of collective spaces of care (such as day centres) (Barnes, 2012); and, third, the everyday realities of their lives, and what they want to achieve balanced with a sense of what is possible (Vincent, 2010). This 'placed' understanding and collaborative working relationship with people with learning disabilities is obvious, but, at the same time, radical. In shifting and broadening the discourse from 'what services do people need?' to 'what are the components of a good life?' (Bartnik and Chalmers, 2007; Johnson *et al.*, 2010), from the assessment of individuals for what practical care they need to thinking about their everyday complex lives, LACs are acting as 'small levers of change' (Bartnik and Chalmers, 2007). In so doing they are challenging the dominant model of person-alised neoliberal welfare, where an individual's relationship with the society is contractual and costed, and are instead focusing on the social and emotional.

> The people we offer support to are individuals that in the main actually know what they want to achieve, they just need a wee bit of guidance to get there. And that's how they view self-directed support, that they're calling the shots, but they need a bit of support to get there and we help bridge the gap, if you like.
>
> (LAC 1, East)

A further challenge to the individualised, monetised model of social care, which devolved social care policy in Scotland is developing and Local Area Co-ordination is facilitating, is the almost complete absence of Direct Payments/Personal Budgets from the debate and practicalities of social care and support. The number of people with learning disabilities in Scotland using a Direct Payment to manage their care and support is very low, compared to almost universal usage in England (Scottish Consortium for Learning Disability, 2012b). The research interviews with LACs supported this national evidence. In 'West', one LAC claimed that only three of 410 adults with learning disabilities (known to the local authority) were in receipt of a Direct Payment. She further commented that the numbers are:

> Very, very low – that's the trend across Scotland pretty much.
>
> (LAC 2, West)

> We actually have very, very few people that have a Direct Payment that they choose to spend as they see fit.
>
> (LAC 1, East)

This should perhaps come as no surprise, given the way in which Direct Payments are described in the National Strategy, as a 'mechanism' (Scottish Government, 2010), rather than as the defining characteristic of personalisation. The National Strategy purposively uses the term 'Self-Directed Support' to broaden the notion of what social care is and is for, that is, beyond individually-received services to the broader context of support within which a person is located. LACs are seem-ingly the people 'on the ground' putting this approach into practice; as Bartnik and Chalmers (2007) put it, LAC is 'about more than the money'. As they state in their formulation of the principles of LAC:

It was decided that it was not necessary to make a direct reference to the LAC role in the co-ordination of direct funding ... Direct funding has proved to be an effective support strategy within the LAC framework ... however, [it] is viewed as an adjunct to family and community-based supports rather than as the primary solution to meeting needs.

(2007: 26–27)

The minor role of Direct Payments in the co-productive work of LACs is of increasing significance as severe funding cuts are made to central and local government budgets. The 'eligibility criteria' used to assess whether an individual is deemed to be in need of social care are being tightened in all local authorities in Scotland (and across the UK), so that many people with a so-called 'moderate' learning disability are no longer judged to be in need of financial support, and funding is concentrated on those in 'severe' and 'critical' need.

A lot of the people we work with would not be people that would necessarily meet the social work [eligibility] criteria.

(LAC 2, West)

Unless you are [in] severe or critical [need], you won't get social work support due to cuts and stuff.

(LAC 1, West)

As Hall and McGarrol (2012) argue, there are an increasing number of people with learning disabilities who are no longer entitled to social care funding, and are also unable to support themselves through paid employment. This expanding 'third space' generates difficulties for many, as they increasingly rely on family support and limited provision of local voluntary organisations (*Guardian*, 2013). But more positively, I wish to argue, this new space is also generative of opportunities for alternative forms, relations and spaces of care and support. LACs were conceived by Bartnik in the late 1980s in a context of reduced state funding, and the need to build alternative sources of community-based support, and as such operate beyond the regulatory system of assessments for eligibility of care. As the Scottish government (2008) stated in its 'National Guidance' for LAC: 'The local co-ordination approach is not based on entitlement to services ... [It] is a way for people currently beyond the reach of the formal service system to access support, and a way of building people's capacity to identify what would better meet their needs.' As the LACs interviewed commented, they work beyond the system of assessment, engaging with people known and unknown to the local authority, and the support offered operates in an increasingly non-economic sphere.

We effectively work as a broker, although no money changes hands, just to explore options for people and support them to look at something different.

(LAC 1, East)

We're more of a preventative role, so we should complement social work in that we get in there early on. We do work, we build people's confidence, we build up people's capacity to become active members of the community, so hopefully they shouldn't ever need social work because they're in a position to deal with any problems as they come up, or they've got us for that extra little bit of assistance and support.

(LAC 1, West)

LACs, through working co-productively at a range of scales, with individuals and families, and with local organisations and agencies, understand people with learning disabilities as being placed in a series of contexts and, in doing so, bridge the development of an ethical way of working with individuals and families. This involves 'foregrounding social relationships of mutuality and trust' (Lawson, 2007: 3) with the building of a possible local ethics of place. LACs are very much defined by their 'local' tag; physically located in places, they almost always live in the areas in which they work and one of the principles of Local Area Co-ordination is to 'contribute to building inclusive communities through partnership and collaboration with individuals and families, local organisations and the broader community' (Bartnik and Chalmers, 2007: 26). Their modus operandi is to place the needs of individuals within the range of contexts, by looking around and beyond into the local community; with the aspirations of those they work with in their minds, LACs over time build working relationships with formal and informal agencies: day centres, Job Centres, Citizens Advice Bureaux, GP surgeries, the Social Work Department of the local authority, local organisations, community groups, voluntary organisations, church congregations and others, including employers. This development work can help access services and open up opportunities for people with learning disabilities and, of greater significance, place people with disabilities in the socio-cultural landscape of the local area, weaving them into the fabric of mainstream 'normality'. The LACs emphasised the importance of connecting people into social relationships and spaces in the places in which they lived, deepening their sense of belonging and, over time, transforming understandings of people with learning disabilities.

We have one LAC who's been working concentrating on a project for young people [with learning disabilities] to enable them to really develop friendships, build confidence, access social opportunities.

(LAC 1, East)

Getting people involved in community activities, or any activities they want to do – employment, education, whatever.

(LAC 1, West)

Through their extensive local contacts, LACs can 'broker' opportunities for the many people with learning disabilities. For some, admittedly a small number, this could be in paid employment (still seen as the key measure of social inclusion).

We can make in-roads to ensuring that people get opportunities to experience work and all the benefits that come along with that ... We're very conscious that the Scottish Government wants to ensure that individuals aren't marginalised and if you want work, let's support you to do that.

(LAC 1, East)

They can help individuals to access the workplace and, once in employment, support the development of key skills, such as independent travel, or through the support of a 'job coach' to work alongside them.

If someone has not had a job before, there is a period where they have to learn ... It took me two years to show him what work was, that you had to go at a certain time, you have to commit yourself to being there.

(LAC, Central)

However, LACs are very realistic about the prospects of sustained and paid employment. A key role is to balance expectations of individuals and families (encouraged by Scottish government statements about the importance of employment to secure social inclusion, and the promise of employment opportunities for all; most recently stated in the new learning disability strategy, Scottish Government, 2013: 94), and the very difficult prospects for people with learning disabilities in employment. The proportion estimated to be in paid employment is estimated to be between 6.4 and 12 per cent, compared to 48 per cent for all disabled people, and 75 per cent for non-disabled people (Department of Health, 2011). A far more promising option is to think beyond paid employment to a wider range of 'work' opportunities, i.e. volunteering, work placements, and other valued contributions within local communities, for example, environmental work and creative arts. I wish to argue that, in fact, a broader conceptualisation of a 'work' role can be hugely beneficial for people with learning disabilities and local communities (and wider society). If people are participating in a wide range of activities, for example, informal caring, environmental activities and community development, beyond the mainstream economy, then they can both gain work-related and everyday life skills and build confidence and self-esteem and wider community valuing.

We enable them to really develop friendships, build confidence, access social opportunities ... be valued and make a contribution. We make sure people out there are using ordinary places and taking part in things you and I do.

(LAC 1, East)

This presence in mainstream spaces and networks – streets, public spaces, shops, voluntary organisations, creative arts centres, churches and so on – secures a valued and meaningful presence for people with learning disabilities in local areas. It might not quite be what local people expect and they may encounter people with learning disabilities in everyday places and spaces, but the gentle provocation of being there in front of people on a daily basis can help to challenge dominant views of what being a (learning) disabled person means.

> People out there in the wider community need to see at first hand, need to experience, need to engage with individuals that are different, whatever their difference may be, and we go some way to sort of breaking down that barrier by making sure that people are out there using ordinary places and taking part in things that you and I do.
>
> (LAC 1, East)

LACs are building what Gibson-Graham (2003) has described as a 'local ethics of care'; that is, through their active co-productive and place-based work with people with learning disabilities, LACs are transforming, albeit gradually and unevenly, the meaning and the landscape of care and support.

Conclusion

This chapter has reflected on how devolution and a particularly progressive form of localism are transforming social care policy-making and practice in Scotland. Commodified personalisation, the dominant model of neoliberal welfare, has been effectively rejected, and a collective, community-based and ethically-informed provision of care and support developed. The chapter has focused upon the co-productive, networked and locally-focused practice of LACs, building what I have referred to as a 'local ethics of care' based on mutuality and trust, centred in community-scale collective spaces and relationships. LACs can both support and strengthen the family-and-friends-centred everyday lives of people with learning disabilities *and* deepen and broaden the relationships and opportunities within the communities in which they live. The proactive, innovative and place-based practices of LACs connect people with learning disabilities into familiar and unfamiliar spaces and activities, improving self-esteem and social presence. Importantly, it is the doing of activities by people with learning disabilities in mainstream local spaces, rather than simply being present, which makes all the difference. Through working co-productively with an LAC (and with support from family, friends and others), a person with a learning disability can generate both feelings of belonging and social valuing for themselves *and* challenge normative (and commonly negative) understandings of the role, status and value of people with (learning) disabilities in local communities (Hall, 2013; Mee and Wright, 2009).

It is important to strike three cautionary notes first, information gathered from LACs (e.g. Scottish Consortium for Learning Disability, 2012c) indicates how in the current funding crisis many are spending most of their time finding ways through the maze of care, support and benefits for people with learning disabilities, and much less time on the arguably more important role of community engagement, threatening the significant potential socio-cultural impact of their work; second, Local Area Co-ordination is not centrally placed in the new Scottish government learning disability strategy, *The keys to life*, which promises an 'outcomes-focused' review of its role in 2014, raising a question mark over its continued existence (Scottish Government, 2013); third, some local authorities are considering reducing the provision of LACs as part of responses to current budget cuts. It is therefore essential to continually make the case for the crucial role that LACs play in helping people with learning disabilities to negotiate the many challenges of everyday life and to pursue a range of opportunities in local areas. However, it is perhaps even more important to highlight and celebrate how the practice of an ethic of care by LACs with people with learning disabilities can both lead to the development of a model of care and caring to challenge the individualism and commodification of social care dominant in so many neoliberal welfare states *and* through an emphasis on building social relationships of trust and mutuality, map out ways of negotiating social and cultural differences within local communities.

References

Barnes, M 2012, *Care in everyday life: an ethic of care in practice*, Policy Press, Bristol.

Bartnik, E and Chalmers, R 2007, 'It's about more than the money: Local Area Co-ordination supporting people with disabilities' in S Hunter and P Ritchie (eds), *Co-production and personalisation in social care*, Jessica Kingsley Publishers, London, pp. 19–38.

Braidotti, R 2012, 'Nomadic ethics' in D Smith and H Somers-Hall (eds), *The Cambridge companion to Deleuze*, Cambridge University Press, Cambridge, pp. 170–197.

Community Care 2012a, *Councils to deny social care support to all but most needy*, accessed 1 May 2013, www.communitycare.co.uk/Articles/15/09/2010/115321/councils-to-deny-social-care-support-to-all-but-most-needy.htm.

Community Care 2012b, *Expert guide to direct payments, personal budgets and individual budgets*, accessed 1 May 2013, www.communitycare.co.uk/Articles/25/07/2012/102669/direct-payments-personal-budgets-and-individual-budgets.htm.

Conradson, D 2011, 'Care and caring' in V del Casino, M Thomas, P Cloke and R Panelli (eds), *A companion to social geography*, Wiley-Blackwell, Chichester, pp. 454–471.

Department for Communities and Local Government 2011, *The Localism Act*, accessed 22 February 2013, www.communities.gov.uk/localgovernment/decentralisation/localismbill/.

Department of Health 2011, *Increasing the numbers of people with learning disabilities in employment*, Department of Health, London.

Featherstone, D, Ince, A, MacKinnon, D, Strauss, K and Cumbers, A 2012, 'Progressive localism and the construction of political alternatives', *Area*, vol. 37, no. 2, pp. 177–182.

Gibson-Graham, J K 2003, 'An ethics of the local', *Rethinking Marxism*, vol. 15, no. 1, pp. 49–74.

Guardian 2013, '"It's like part of your family has gone missing": austerity is forcing community organisations that offer vital services to vulnerable people to close their doors', 15 May, p. 32.

Hall, E 2011, 'Shopping for support: personalisation and the new spaces and relations of commodified care for people with learning disabilities', *Social and Cultural Geography*, vol. 12, no. 6, pp. 589–603.

Hall, E 2013, 'Making, gifting and performing belonging: creative arts and people with learning disabilities', *Environment and Planning A*, vol. 45, no. 2, pp. 244–262.

Hall, E and Kearns, R 2001, 'Making space for the "intellectual" in geographies of disability', *Health and Place*, vol. 7, no. 3, pp. 237–246.

Hall, E and McGarrol, S 2012, 'Bridging the gap between employment and social care for people with learning disabilities: Local Area Co-ordination and in-between spaces of social inclusion', *Geoforum*, vol. 43, pp. 1276–1286.

Hatton, C, Waters, J, Duffy, S, Senker, J, Crosby, N, Poll, C, Tyson, A, O'Brien, J and Towell, D 2008, *A report on In Control's second phase 2005–07*, In Control, London.

Hughes, B, McKie, L, Hopkins, D and Watson, N 2005, 'Loves labour's lost: feminism, the disabled people's movement and an ethic of care', *Sociology*, vol. 39, no. 2, pp. 259–275.

Hunter, S and Ritchie, P 2007, 'Introduction: with, not to: models of co-production in social welfare', in S Hunter and P Ritchie (eds), *Co-production and personalisation in social care*, Jessica Kingsley Publishers, London, pp. 9–18.

Johnson, K, Walmsley, J and Wolfe, M 2010, *People with intellectual disabilities: towards a good life*, Policy Press, Bristol.

Keating, M 2005, 'Policy divergence and convergence in Scotland under devolution', *Regional Studies*, vol. 39, no. 4, pp. 453–463.

Lawson, V 2007, 'Geographies of care and responsibility', *Annals of the Association of American Geographers*, vol. 97, no. 1, pp. 1–11.

Levitas, R 2012, 'The just's umbrella: austerity and the big society in coalition and beyond', *Critical Social Policy*, vol. 32, no. 3, pp. 320–342.

Manthorpe, J, Hindes, J, Martineau, S, Cornes, M, Ridley, J, Spandler, H, Rosengard, A, Hunter, S, Little, S and Gray, B 2011, *Self-directed support: a review of the barriers and facilitators*, Scottish Government Social Research, Edinburgh.

Massey, D 2004, 'Geographies of responsibility', *Geografiska Annaler*, vol. 86B, no. 1, pp. 5–18.

Mee, K and Wright, S 2009, 'Geographies of belonging', *Environment and Planning A*, vol. 41, pp. 772–779.

Metzel, D and Philo, C 2005, 'Introduction to theme section on geographies of intellectual disability: "outside the participatory mainstream"?', *Health and Place*, vol. 11, no. 2, pp. 77–85.

Mooney, G and Scott, G 2012, *Social justice and social policy in Scotland*, Policy Press, Bristol.

Morris, J 1997, 'Care or empowerment? A disability rights perspective', *Social Policy and Administration*, vol. 31, no. 1, pp. 54–60.

Power, A 2008, 'Caring for independent lives: geographies of caring for young adults with intellectual disabilities', *Social Science and Medicine*, vol. 67, pp. 834–843.

Raco, M 2009, 'From expectations to aspirations: state modernisation, urban policy, and the existential politics of welfare in the UK', *Political Geography*, vol. 28, pp. 436–444.

Reinders, H 2000, *The future of the disabled in liberal society: an ethical analysis*, University of Notre Dame Press, Indiana.

Ridley, J, Spandler, H, Rosengard, A, Little, S, Cornes, M, Manthorpe, J, Hunter, S, Kinder, T and Gray, B 2011, *Evaluation of self-directed support test sites in Scotland*, Scottish Government Social Research, Edinburgh.

Scottish Consortium for Learning Disability 2012a, *Local Area Co-ordinators*, accessed 1 May 2013, www.scld.org.uk/local-area-co-ordination/contacts-list.

Scottish Consortium for Learning Disability 2012b, *Statistics release, adults with learning disabilities*, SCLD, Glasgow.

Scottish Consortium for Learning Disability 2012c, *Local area co-ordination national gathering January 2012 report*, SCLD, Glasgow.

Scottish Executive 2000, *The same as you? A review of services for people with learning disabilities*, The Stationery Office, Edinburgh.

Scottish Government 2008, *National guidance on the implementation of local area co-ordination*, Scottish Government, Edinburgh.

Scottish Government 2010, *Self-directed support: a national strategy for Scotland*, Scottish Government, Edinburgh.

Scottish Government 2012, *Self-directed support (Direct Payments) Scotland 2012*, National Statistics for Scottish Government, Edinburgh.

Scottish Government 2013, *The keys to life: improving quality of life for people with learning disabilities*, Scottish Government, Edinburgh.

Scottish Government and COSLA 2007, *Concordat*, Scottish Government and COSLA, Edinburgh.

Tronto, J 1993, *Moral boundaries: a political argument for an ethic of care*, Routledge, London.

Vincent, A 2010, 'Local Area Co-ordination: an exploration of practice developments in Western Australia and Northern Ireland', *Practice: Social Work in Action*, vol. 22, no. 4, pp. 203–216.

Westwood, A 2011, 'Localism, social capital and the "Big Society"', *Local Economy*, vol. 26, no. 8, pp. 690–701.

9 Institutionalised lives and exclusion from spaces of intimacy for people with learning difficulties

Andrea Hollomotz and Alan Roulstone

Introduction

Other chapters in this book have helpfully documented the fact that disabled people are at times excluded from public spaces, resulting in many spending a disproportionate amount of their time in segregated social care and domestic settings or when in public space facing environmental and economic barriers to both 'being' and 'doing'. This chapter explores the less well-trodden territory of the lack of private space and sexual citizenship for some disabled people, most especially those with learning difficulties (referred to as intellectual disabilities in many countries and as learning disabilities by official governmental authorities in England), by looking at denial of intimacy in group home contexts. We will do this by contextualising the analyses in the broader literature on space, power and citizenship. The chapter begins by providing background and context from the broader literature on power and the regulation of space and intimacy. It then provides a macro-level policy picture of disability policy and intimacy and then more specific policy appraisal of group homes. The second half of this chapter draws on in-depth interviews with people with learning difficulties and focus groups with a self-advocacy group, which will illustrate these themes. The chapter concludes that the right to privacy must be formally acknowledged and enforced in social policy and in enabling practice.

The social regulation of space

The chapter applies a sociological definition to the concept of 'private sphere'. The term is used not merely to describe privately occupied spaces opposed to those that are publicly accessible. 'Privacy' implies autonomy to adopt a 'backstage identity' (Goffman, 1959), to adopt more 'relaxed' behaviour patterns and to engage in activities, including those of a sexual nature, which would not be desirable in public spheres. Normative notions of space, intimacy and privacy are however not universal and timeless. Aries' classic study of the family through history notes that childhood and the rights to personal space only became widespread in eighteenth-century Europe (Aries, 1988). Ulanowicz picks up the story in noting:

The rise of the family Aries writes, was the consequence of a general movement in Western society from sociability to privacy. Before the 18th century
noble families lived in 'great houses' in which space was shared between
children and adults and servants and masters.

(Ulanowicz, n.d.)

Privacy was then seen as a contrast to undifferentiated social space as well as
greater delineations of space and privacy within a family. Such affordances of
one's own space represent not simply space and privacy, but are symbolic of changing power distributions within families in Western society.

In contemporary Western official and lay accounts of adulthood it is assumed
that space, choices and citizenship are intimately linked. Independence, self-
determination and lifestyle choices are epitomised in images of getting a place of
one's own and one of the first symbolic freedoms is to embrace the affordances
of privacy and sexual choices (Chapman and Hockey, 2013). However, such normative constructions do not usually account for the assumptions and freedoms
afforded to people with learning difficulties, for whom different social norms and
assumptions seem to apply.

Pre-existing assumptions about learning difficulty have tended to err on the side
of constructing sex and sexual choices for people with learning difficulties as secondary to protection from risk and the effects of 'innate vulnerability' (Roulstone
et al. in Roulstone and Mason-Bish, 2012). Sexual activity and desire, rather than
be seen as situated on a 'normal' spectrum of adult choice and expression, continue to be constructed as risky, deviant or asexual (as characterises childhood
pre-puberty) (O'Callaghan and Murphy, 2007). This is evident even where capacity is not at issue (O'Callaghan and Murphy, 2004).

Whilst we need to be careful to avoid Western-centric interpretations of family forms and power (Ozaki, 1900), we can reasonably assert that power, space,
control and broader social values are intimately linked. At the intersection of the
public world of planners and policy-makers and the personal world of family,
friends and neighbours, the home is a site in which key social and personal values
can be examined (Chapman and Hockey, 2013: xi). Indeed, many of the early
struggles by disabled people for civil rights were spatial in nature, with activists
and academics questioning the 'inevitable' institutionalisation and infantilising of
disabled people (Finkelstein, 1980; Hunt, 1966). Anthropologically we can see
the continued enforced collective institutionalisation as running counter to the
spatial rights afforded even able-bodied children by the eighteenth and nineteenth
centuries. Peter Townsend's powerful foreword to Paul Hunt's collected essays on
stigma sums up the links between being 'put away' and broader constructions of
the problem of disability:

They [disabled people] realize how widespread are feelings of protectiveness,
superiority, aloofness and even revulsion towards them. Ordinary people
often expect them to become passive and compliant independents, an isolated
category of the pitied who are thrust out of sight at home or in institutions,

no wonder they write of the bitterness and frustration involved in playing the role of invalid.

(Hunt, 1966: 2)

The social regulation of intimacy

Weeks' (2012) elaborate outline of *The regulation of sexuality since 1800* demonstrates that whether and which sexual behaviours are perceived to be 'normal' is continually re-defined and specific to particular points in time and social contexts. For instance, at the beginning of the modern era sexual acts other than penetration were likely to be a 'more collective, semi-"public" affair – even masturbation, let alone the broad range of nonpenetrative acts of petting, fondling, bundling and the like' (McKeon, 2005: 272). However, through time, sexual intimacy has been increasingly rule-bound and hetero-normative. From the late nineteenth century sex and sexuality have been closely bound up and powerful cultural messages from the church, state and academy have presented essentially cultural views on 'right' sexualities as new moral sciences. Science itself has helped cement the binary notions of healthy sexual appetites that align unproblematically to wider notions of normativity.

A further example is the construction of female sexuality. Havelock Ellis, whom Weeks (2012: 191) describes as 'the greatest of the British writers on sexuality who emerged at the end of the nineteenth century', assumed that female sexuality was secondary and essentially responsive to male desire. Jackson contends that Ellis' work made a significant contribution towards the eroticisation of female oppression, as to him: 'heterosexual intercourse was essentially a re-enactment of primitive, animal courtship; the male sexual urge was essentially an urge to conquer and the female sexual urge an urge to be conquered' (Jackson, 1987: 57). We see that by the late nineteenth century, strong views as to sex, sexuality and normative parameters had been graced with 'scientific' and thus unchallengeable assumptions. Although Weeks does not explore explicitly disability and sexual drives and intimacy, his broader thesis is clear that hetero-normativity and biology create the foundations on which intimacy is judged. In this way, disabled people represent a threat to these norms of 'healthy' biology and sex.

Space, disability policy and intimacy

As this book seeks to explore the intersection of space, disability and policy, it is worth reflecting for a while on attempts to underpin rights to sexual citizenship in legislation and policy in England. Legislation is now firmly in place to support reasonable access to the workplace, leisure and civic spaces under the Disability Discrimination Act (Lawson, 2008). Part M of the Building Regulations (Imrie, 2004) aims to establish good physical access to non-domestic buildings that afford minimal access standards. These laws, and the policies and codes of practice that underpin them, are however premised on notions of gaining access to space, as opposed to certain key freedoms and inclusions once there. As such they equate to the notion of integration as opposed to inclusion (Vislie, 2003); measures where a person with a learning difficulty can be spatially integrated but where there remains a reaffirmation of categorical differences between disabled and non-disabled people.

Statements on choice and rights to intimacy for people with learning difficulties then are contained in more general policy statements that aim to foster attitude change which better supports choices for disabled people. For disabled adults, key policy documents point to the need to foster independence, choice and selfhood. For example, under the previous Labour government, *Valuing people* (DoH, 2001), *Independence, wellbeing and choice* (DoH, 2005), *Our health, our care, our say* (DoH, 2006) each drove home the message of choices and fulfilled lives for disabled adults, themes that were also picked up by the current Coalition government (Her Majesty's Government, 2012). However, there is also scope for cynicism. Fyson warns that such policy is 'sold under the comforting banners of "independence", "choice" and "control" in order to mask the less palatable reality of budget cuts' (Fyson, 2009: 19).

Furthermore, such policy messages are helpful if one already has a home, relationship and therefore spaces of intimacy. More significantly, however, these laws and policy papers do not offer substantial rights to intimacy. Of note, where *Independence, wellbeing and choice* explores relationships and gets close to substantiating choices it curiously veers towards managing 'complex relationships' and is some distance away from a more affirmative construction that would better support sexual choice-making:

> It can include practical assistance to help individuals overcome barriers to inclusion, such as supported entry into work for an individual with a mental health problem, a personal assistant to enable a disabled person to lead a full and active life or supporting a person with a learning disability to play a full part in their local community. It can include support in managing complex relationships and emotional distress.
>
> (DoH, 2005: 24)

Valuing people, a key White Paper focused entirely on learning difficulty, does however offer the basic mindset and value framework to begin to translate choices into previously taboo areas such as sexual intimacy:

> People with learning disabilities are often socially isolated. Helping people sustain friendships is consistently shown as being one of the greatest challenges faced by learning disability services. Good services will help people with learning disabilities develop opportunities to form relationships, including ones of a physical and sexual nature. It is important that people can receive accessible sex education and information about relationships and contraception.
>
> (DoH, 2001: 88)

However, even *Valuing people* makes very few detailed references to sexual choices or intimacy and the specific forms these might take. Indeed more references are made in the document to the risk of people with learning difficulties being victims of sexual abuse (DoH, 2001: 31, 32, 101). The three-year consultation about the future of 'learning disability' services, *Valuing people now* (DoH, 2009) makes no references to sex or intimacy in its consultation outline. The question of sexual rights, freedoms and choices still seems some distance away from the realities of social 'care' policy in England. The connection between the choices agenda, as laid out above, and life in group homes, also seems to have been very limited in policy and practice terms. The spatial implications are twofold – first, that spaces of intimacy are not dealt with substantively in most adult social care policy, and second, space and choice seems not to extend its reach into collective living contexts such as group homes.

The small group 'home' in England

At the beginning of the twentieth century, people with learning difficulties were included under the umbrella term 'mental defectives'. Eugenicists believed this population was reproducing 'excessively', thus 'threatening' the national heritage of intelligence. Consequently, the 1913 Mental Deficiency Act enacted segregation in asylums (Weeks, 2012). Separation of the sexes was assumed to prevent sexual activity and thus the passing of 'defective' genetic material to the next generation.

Besides acting as a measure for population control, institutions fulfilled two paradoxically contrasting purposes: on the one hand, they were seen as protecting society from individuals who were seen as deviant and dangerous. On the other hand, the aim was to provide a safe and stimulating environment for people categorised as having a disability (Walmsley, 2005). All aspects of life, such as sleeping, eating, work, education and leisure activities, were conducted within institutions, which were characterised by barriers to social intercourse with the outside world, such as locked doors, high walls and barbed wire (Goffman, 1961). The agency of inmates was diminished through the control of their use of space and activities, which were usually tightly scheduled and conducted in large batches (Valentine, 2001). In the last quarter of the twentieth century the way in which services for people with learning difficulties were provided changed towards predominantly community-based provisions. However, Philo and Parr argue that deinstitutionalisation has resulted in a 'fragmenting of asylums' into smaller facilities:

> the dispersal of the asylum has simply resulted in the opening of smaller but equally isolating places ... spinning a torn web of deinstitutionalised but in many respects still 'institutional' geographies across the city and beyond. The purpose of the traditional institution (in its role to confine, monitor, correct or cure) is arguably still apparent, although now operating through different medical, social and legal apparatuses.
>
> (Philo and Parr, 2000: 514)

Today, the majority of people with learning difficulties in England live in private homes (roughly 40 per cent live with family or friends and 16 per cent live in a tenancy). The second largest group of people with learning difficulties live in formal support settings (approximately 20 per cent live in registered care 'homes' and around 16 per cent live in supported living arrangements) (Emerson *et al.*, 2012). The remainder of this chapter examines whether and to what extent Philo and Parr's (2000) claim applies to the ways in which spaces for intimacy are organised within modern support settings for people with learning difficulties.

For O'Brien (1994), the word home has specific connotations. It does not merely refer to any kind of residential arrangement. A home must provide individuals with security of place through tenancy or ownership, control over the home and the necessary support for living there. Annison (2000) adds that a home does not merely serve to meet basic needs (e.g. shelter), but that it is also central to the fulfilment of emotional and relationship needs. A home can provide individuals with a sense of belonging. It gives them a means of self-expression and an opportunity to take on responsibility (Chapman and Hockey, 2013).

As indicated earlier, in England, we distinguish between residential care 'homes' and supported living. The latter should usually be small group houses, ideally of no more than three people and they are not registered as care or nursing 'homes' (Emerson *et al.*, 2001). Residents should hold their own tenancies and are thus assumed to have more control over their environment than those living in residential care. While supported living settings can potentially provide tenancies, they are often set up and run by a specific care agency, which acts to limit the control that tenants themselves have over the set up and running of the 'home', where and who they live with and who provides support.

On the whole, compared to institutional provisions, community based settings achieve better results in terms of quality of life and social skills (O'Brien *et al.*, 2001), community participation, contact with family and friends and overall satisfaction with the service (Mansell, 2006). However, to what extent can such establishments be considered 'homes' in a conventional sense?

> The home is not just a three-dimensional structure, a shelter, but it is also a matrix of social relations … and has wider symbolic and ideological meanings … Traditionally, the home has been constructed as a private space in opposition to the public space of the world of work.
>
> (Valentine, 2001: 63)

In geographical terms, the twenty-first-century residential group establishment poses a paradox, because it is both a private space, where residents spend their leisure and relaxation time, and a public space, where staff work to support such leisure and relaxation (Lindegaard and Brodersen, 2010). Due to low rates of employment and lack of mobility, disabled people are likely to spend more time at 'home' than non-disabled people (Hamer, 2005), which increases the significance of this space in their lives (Hemingway, 2011).

Levinson (2010) adds that, even in the absence of paid employment within the group 'home', residents, too, continuously 'work'. He asserts that the explicit aim of such establishments is to foster 'independence', a concept he appears to define uncritically, in line with dominant Western ideals. Morris describes such an approach as 'associated with the ability to do things for oneself, to be self-supporting, self-reliant. Those who cannot do things for themselves are assumed to be unable to control their lives' (Morris, 1993: 22–3). He explains that, in a community residence, 'the goal is not independence per se but its pursuit, and for individuals unable to achieve independence in any conventional sense, this pursuit is endless' (Levinson, 2010: 103). Residents' 'work', therefore, entails taking on 'their own selves as ongoing projects of independence' (Levinson, 2010: 249), while staff support this process. Consequently, in such settings the distinction between 'work' and 'home' is much more complex than Valentine's (2001) more general definition suggests.

The study

The second half of this chapter draws on two studies exploring sexual choices in the lives of people with learning difficulties. The first study consisted of four focus group discussions which were conducted with 15 self-advocates during a service user consultation on local sex and relationship policy. The group consisted of eight women and seven men, all of whom were white British and have learning difficulties. During our discussions, self-advocates identified lack of privacy in residential group settings as a particular concern they wished to address. After we were informed at local level that this could not be resolved via immediate policy, we decided to share our concerns with a wider audience (Hollomotz and The Speakup Committee, 2009). The second study was a three-year research project consisting of semi-structured interviews with 12 men and 17 women with learning difficulties and participant observations which explored the social, sexual and leisure lives, 'vulnerabilities' and risks of adults with learning difficulties (Hollomotz, 2011).

The ages of participants across both projects ranged from early twenties to late sixties. Respondents in the interviews had labels of 'mild' to 'moderate' learning difficulties. About half had additional impairment labels, such as physical impairments, epilepsy and 'Autistic spectrum' labels. Furthermore, half lived with their parents or other family members. About a quarter lived in residential group settings and another quarter lived on their own or with a partner. To enable the reader to distinguish between respondents from this study and the focus group based study, respondents' pseudonyms will be followed by (INT) if they arise from the interview based study and (FG) if they arise from focus group discussions. Furthermore, this chapter focuses mostly on accounts and debates that are relevant for formal group living. However, it will at times include examples provided by adults who live with family carers or of those who use day services.

Sex, privacy and the group 'home'

Privacy is taken to mean 'the state or condition of being alone, undisturbed, or free from public attention, as a matter of choice or right' and 'freedom from interference or intrusion' (OED online, 2012). Furthermore,

> [p]rivacy permits people to share intimacies and ideas on their own terms, and thus establish those mutual reciprocal relinquishments of the self that underlie the relations of love, friendship and trust … The right to privacy is thus an inescapable aspect of our humanity.
>
> (Krattenmarker cited in Silver, 1997: 43)

This section is broken down into three sub-sections. First, the extent to which privacy is realised in respondents' bedrooms is considered. Second, four case studies, which highlight how intimacy of people with learning difficulties is at times supervised, are discussed. Third, the final part exposes an adverse effect of restricted privacy: the marginalisation of sexual activity into isolated semi-private spaces indoors or outdoors.

Seeking privacy in the bedroom

Findings from the study of group homes suggested that while divisions between allocated spaces for each resident (e.g. 'Sarah's room') may limit the geographies of the residents (e.g. Tom will not enter Sarah's room), staff remained free to float from one space to another. Whether and to what extent they respect this private space of residents will depend on individual staff and the rules within each setting. Rachel (INT, early thirties) complained that some of the staff do not knock before entering her room: 'Like [staff] opened the door: "Are you ready? Are you dressed smart? Are you decent?" … didn't knock on the door! They didn't! They just walk in! March in!'.

Similar examples were cited by the self-advocates. Shared bedrooms exaggerate this sense of invasion, as individuals are rarely alone in their room. One of the self-advocates remembers how it felt to share until recently: 'I wasn't my own boss then. I didn't have my own space. I could not be private at all.' Creating private space for a sexual relationship or for masturbation becomes much more difficult. Perhaps it would be less surprising to find residents who are placed in such an unusual setting, when measured on contemporary 'norms' (unrelated adults who are not in a romantic relationship sharing a bedroom), act in ways that are considered 'less appropriate' within the wider cultural context, such as masturbating whilst another person who is not a sexual partner is in the room. In settings where bedrooms (shared or not) do furthermore not have locks, the bathroom will be the only space where individuals who can mobilise without assistance may seek some refuge from intrusion. Those who have their own bedrooms and are seeking to use this space for intimacy with a partner are often confronted by further hurdles. For example, all of the self-advocates who lived in group 'homes' slept in single beds, but as some single beds are very narrow, there was not enough space to share with another person. Even if a couple would be prepared to squeeze in together, sharing a single bed would then contradict the policies enforced by the residential establishment.

Rosenblatt (2006) explains that, for many people, the shared couple bed is a place of great safety, security, comfort and trust. He describes how some people use routines around the couple bed to distract themselves from upsetting, painful, worrisome or frightening thoughts. For instance, he cites the example of a woman who is unable to go to sleep at times, unless her partner comes to bed and reads to her. Rosenblatt further asserts that, due to the competing demands of modern life arising from work, leisure and consumption, which make it difficult for a couple to have much contact, 'it is in the sleep situation that the couple connection is symbolised' (Rosenblatt, 2006: 11). Sharing a bed does therefore strengthen a relationship.

A prerequisite for bed sharing is the ability to bring a chosen sexual partner to one's bedroom. Even after a person has successfully negotiated any capacity assessments (as discussed later on), their hopes are likely to be crushed by the service provider's regulations, which often prohibit 'visitors' from entering bedrooms unsupervised, unless they are staff, professionals or blood relatives, which, in line with 'fire and safety regulations', was the main reason why the self-advocacy group's request to enforce privacy in group 'homes' via the local sex and relationship policy was rejected. For example, Betty (FG), one of the self-advocates, noted:

> My boyfriend once went to my bedroom. Staff came and checked on him. They asked: 'What are you doing here?' and told him to leave. (He only came in to drop off a can of pop.)

The following is an extract from the consultation document that was forwarded to the local authority at the time, which sums up part of this request:

> Staff at residential homes should not be allowed to stop a person from having their partner stay overnight. Our residential homes have rules that do not allow another person to stay over. But there should be ways around them. Especially people in long-term relationships are very frustrated. We want to do in our home whatever we like to do. That is what other people do. We want privacy and a right to sexual lives.
>
> (FG)

Similarly, Anna (FG) recalls an incident that happened when she was living in a hostel a couple of years earlier:

> I was in a bedroom with this boy and we were watching the telly. Staff came in and told me off. We weren't doing anything. We were just watching the telly. They misunderstood. They would not allow us to be in his room together after that.

The ultimate and common symbolism for having no delineated intimacy was the absence of locks on people's bedroom doors. Jodie (FG) recalls that, after residents had sought privacy in their bedroom, staff decided to remove the existing locks from the doors.

Supervised intimacy

Consenting adults having to negotiate with another adult, or indeed a whole panel of professionals, whether and in what ways they may be allowed to be intimate with one another, is not an unusual occurrence in learning difficulties services. For instance, one of the authors of this chapter previously described their puzzlement at an adult protection case conference, where professionals scrutinised the intimate sexual behaviours of a couple who resided in a small group establishment. Adult protection proceedings were initiated after they were observed being intimate in their living room: 'They had both been fully dressed when the man put his head between the woman's breasts' (Hollomotz, 2011: 13). A social worker felt that the woman had been sexually exploited.

Some readers might think it strange that this couple displayed such explicit sexual behaviour in front of another person. One could suggest that they should have delayed this until they were alone. An explanation for why they had not done so could be that, due to their learning difficulties, the couple lacked privacy awareness. This gives rise to a number of further concerns: if the couple lack privacy awareness, how much do they know about sex and relationships? Do they indeed have the capacity to consent to this sexual behaviour?

However, this approach could pose a risk of diagnostic overshadowing (Reiss *et al.*, 1982), as it attributes the observed unusual behaviour to a person's impairment, which closes down avenues for further exploration. An alternative explanation could be that the couple had made a competent judgement. Within a 'home' setting where they were strictly prohibited from visiting each other's bedrooms, the only spaces they had for sexual exploration were communal. In other words, they had learned *not* to seek privacy, as this had been sanctioned in the past. Ryan (INT, late twenties) has a past history of sex offending and as such may be constructed as both *at risk* and *a risk*. As a precautious measure he receives one-to-one supervision at all times. When he first started dating a woman using the same social support agency, his 'risk management plan' prohibited privacy with another 'vulnerable' person. This plan was set out by his legal guardian, the social services authority. For couples such as this, the enforcement of rules that prohibit privacy may *appear* unreasonable if they are not fully explained. Service providers are often faced with competing demands of safeguarding one party, whilst keeping the offending history of the other party confidential, which limits the strength of the explanations that may be given. Under such circumstances it may be argued that the unsuspecting partner is unable to make a fully informed decision about this relationship, which is why risk management strategies may need to be put in place.

However, Ryan's case study also demonstrates that, at least in some instances, the boundaries between freedom and risk may be carefully negotiated in partnership with the couple concerned. At this point it is worth bearing in mind that, in some cases, sexually violent behaviour in men with learning difficulties has been linked to difficulties in establishing adult sexual relationships (Dale 1993, 1994, cited in Allam *et al.*, 1997). This can further justify why the risks and opportunities that may arise from this consenting relationship should be considered holistically.

The risk management plan was eventually revised. The updated version stated that Ryan and his partner can spend time alone in each other's bedroom with the door closed, but not locked. A member of staff must knock on the door every five minutes and await a positive response from both parties. The support worker would only open the door if one person would ask for help or not answer. They will return five minutes later to check again. This arrangement worked well for a number of months and the distance between intervals was gradually increased to 15 minutes. After the first two case studies focused on supervised intimacies between couples, the subsequent two case studies highlight that masturbation, too, is at times supervised and monitored. Norman (INT, early thirties) lives with his dad and his dad's partner. He has learned that masturbation should take place in his bedroom. When he wants to masturbate, he announces that he does not want to be disturbed. Whilst dad and partner will usually enter Norman's room without knocking, he will remain undisturbed after he asked for privacy:

> In house … my bedroom. Sometimes I do it. In my bedroom … cause I've got pictures [of glamour models] on the walls. So that's my private bits. Yeah. I do. I've got some pants, to do it in … and then they [dad or partner] wash them. And then get fresh, so it's easy.

Norman has learned that context and space impact on whether or not masturbation is acceptable:

> When outside … That's rude, cause if they do it, police could lock me up … That's naughty … Dad says: 'Keep a good hiding for it.' That's naughty. Should not do it outside. Do it where I do it. In a flat or house.

Rachel (INT, early thirties) ended a sexual relationship a few months prior to the interview. When she confided in her mother that she misses sex, she bought her a vibrator:

> I bought it for a reason, cause eh, my mum bought it me. Me mum said to me to use it, because I've got [erogenous] spots. So that means I have to clean it. Morning and night. And then, if I've got any spots, put this gel onto it and then, use it … It's like a pear shape. It makes a funny, funny noise … Like, vibrator. I got one of them … And I can't say it in front of [fellow resident].

Rachel lives with one other woman. Her fellow resident does not know about the vibrator, but all the staff do. Rachel can keep her vibrator overnight, but it must be locked in the medication cupboard every morning. Staff sign it in and out. This may appear strange to the outside observer. Certainly, in some remote sense, sex may be considered a 'medical need', as it brings with it considerable health benefits (Lindau and Gavrilova, 2010). However, this makes it sound awfully dull and it is not usually the first association that springs to mind. What is more, staff could be said to monitor and control Rachel's sexual appetite, which could act to inhibit Rachel from asking for her vibrator as frequently as she desires it.

Both Norman and Rachel can thus successfully create spaces of intimacy upon request. While the act of asking for such a space could be perceived as potentially humiliating, neither Norman nor Rachel would share such a view. Their accounts are matter-of-fact descriptions. Both seem comfortable and familiar with the level of intrusion they are exposed to, which may either reflect the sensitivity with which the support is provided (all of Rachel's staff are female), or simply the fact that they are used to routine intrusions into their privacy. What all four case studies demonstrate is that privacy does not merely constitute a given physical space, such as a bedroom, but that whether or not this space becomes free from intrusions and is thus permitted to be used for intimacy is determined by further negotiations. Would Rachel be allowed to masturbate in her bedroom at lunchtime?

Escape into semi-private spheres

Some people with learning difficulties who are sexually active are escaping to unsafe locations, not by choice, but by necessity. Lack of privacy forces them to conduct 'their sexual lives outdoors or in semi-private places indoors, such as back staircases or unused rooms' (McCarthy, 1999: 153). Peter (INT, late fifties) explains:

> The only other way is, you can go out, out there. Go outside and you can spend that, have a sexy half hour or, eh, five minutes with your girlfriend, cause, that's what it's known to be. Like I say about this, if the people in the home know … that that's happening … all they probably would have to say is: 'O, eh, you know, don't, you know, don't do that!'.

Sexual activity becomes thus secretive, rushed and less visible. Many of the self-advocates (FG) knew of secluded spaces that were informally known to be 'hotspots' for sexual activity, such as behind a wall in the garden, behind a shed or in the car park. This remoteness is important, as Chantal (INT, early twenties) explains: 'I would find a quiet place first, cause you don't want to do it if, there's like loads of people.' The spaces that are sought out are not primarily chosen for comfort, which is secondary to remoteness, as highlighted by McCarthy's (1999: 154) descriptions of an extreme example:

A woman with learning disabilities offered to show me the caravan she and many others had sex in. I could not believe what I was seeing … it was a wreck, littered with broken glass, filth (including excrement of some kind) and rubbish.

As (Hollomotz and The Speakup Committee, 2009) asserted previously, hasty sexual activity allows little space for negotiations of personal boundaries. Consequently, individuals have limited time to consider whether they consent to a proposed sexual act and to communicate their decision, which places them at risk of sexual violence from their partner. Absence of support can be linked to the fact that, in some learning difficulties settings, sexuality continues to be either 'not a problem, because it is not an issue, or [it] is an issue, because it is seen as a problem' (Shakespeare *et al.*, 1996: 3). Instead of supporting positive sexual expression, people who receive support with a range of other aspects of their social and leisure lives are quite literally left 'out in the cold' (car park, shed or wherever). Such practices contravene the UK's Human Rights Act (Her Majesty's Government, 1998: Article 8(1)) and the UN Convention on the Rights of Persons with Disabilities (United Nations, 2006: Article 22), which protect the right of people with disabilities to respect for private, home and family life.

Conclusions: looking ahead

Residents in group 'homes' may feel as if they are living in a glass house at times, as there are few spaces to hide from the curious gaze of others. If bedrooms are 'off-limits' areas for couples seeking privacy, they may look for escapes in areas in or around their 'home', which are less well monitored. Notions of power and imposed constructions of risk and vulnerability are still very evident in determining normative politics of space, intimacy and choice. Fully deinstitutionalised group living has not yet become reality, as this would mirror the use of space that is commonplace in the community. Bedrooms would usually be used for comfort and leisure, sleep, privacy and sexual exploration. Sheds would be used for the storage of garden tools and not as makeshift escapes.

Many local services in England have developed relationship policies, whilst self and organisational advocacy will each in turn raise expectations amongst people with learning difficulties. This will, over time, impact positively on the experiences of individuals. Nevertheless, those who have written their local policy should not simply put this on a shelf and consider the work done. First, policies will only work if considerable resources, such as staff training and service user awareness-raising, are made available. However, additional facilities and services are required to make implementation a reality. Second, simply having a policy of some sorts will not do. Some guidance may turn out to be vague and therefore less helpful. Other guidance, it may be discovered, may simply not be suitable for a particular service user, whose needs may differ from those that were originally assumed by the writers of the policy. Relationship policies should therefore be open to scrutiny and regularly reviewed and updated.

References

Allam, J, Middleton, D and Browne, K 1997, 'Different clients, different needs? Practice issues in community-based treatment for sex offenders', *Criminal Behaviour and Mental Health*, vol. 7, no. 1, pp. 69–84.

Annison, J E 2000, 'Towards a clearer understanding of the meaning of "home"', *Journal of Intellectual and Developmental Disability*, vol. 25, no. 4, pp. 251–262.

Aries, P 1988, *Centuries of childhood: a social history of family life*, Random House, New York.

Chapman, A and Hockey, J (eds) 2013, *Ideal homes? Social change and domestic life*, Routledge, London.

DoH 2001, *Valuing people: a new strategy for learning disability in the 21st century*, Department of Health, London.

DoH 2005, *Independence, wellbeing and choice: our vision for the future of social care for adults in England*, Department of Health, London.

DoH 2006, *Our health, our care, our say: a new direction for community services*, Department of Health, London.

DoH 2009, *Valuing people now: a new three year strategy for people with learning disabilities. Making it happen for everyone*, Department of Health, London.

Emerson, E, Hatton, C, Robertson, J, Roberts, H, Baines, S, Evison, F and Glover, G 2012, *People with learning disabilities in England 2011*, Improving Health and Lives: Learning Disabilities Observatory, Stockton on Tees.

Emerson, E, Robertson, J, Gregory, N, Hatton, C, Kessissoglou, S, Hallam, A, Järbrink, K, Knapp, M, Netten, A and Noonan Walsh, P 2001, 'Quality and costs of supported living residences and group homes in the United Kingdom', *Am J Ment Retard*, vol. 106, no. 5, pp. 401–415.

Finkelstein, V (1980) *Attitudes and Disabled People*. New York: World Rehabilitation Fund Monograph.

Fyson, R 2009, 'Independence and learning disabilities: why we must also recognize vulnerability', *The Journal of Adult Protection*, vol. 11, no. 3, pp. 18–25.

Goffman, E 1959, *The presentation of self in everyday life*, Anchor, New York.

Goffman, E 1961, *Asylums: essays on the social situation of mental patients and other inmates*, Doubleday, Garden City.

Hamer, R 2005, *House hunting for all: opening up property search systems to disabled people*, Ownership Options in Scotland, Edinburgh.

Hemingway, L 2011, *Disabled people and housing: choices, opportunities and barriers*, Policy Press, Bristol.

Her Majesty's Government 1998, *Statute: Human Rights Act*, HMSO, London.

Her Majesty's Government 2012, *Statute: Health and Social Care Act*, HMSO, London.

Hollomotz, A 2011, *Learning difficulties and sexual vulnerability: a social approach*, Jessica Kingsley Publishers, London.

Hollomotz, A. and The Speakup Committee (2009), '"May we please have sex tonight?" People with learning difficulties pursuing privacy in residential group settings', *British Journal of Learning Disabilities*, vol. 37, no. 2, pp. 91–97.

Hunt, P 1966, *Stigma: the experience of disability*, Geoffrey Chapman, London.

Imrie, R 2004, 'Disability, embodiment and the meaning of home', *Housing Studies*, vol. 19, no. 5, pp. 745–763.

Jackson, M 1987, '"Facts of life" or the eroticisation of women's oppression? Sexology and the social construction of heterosexuality', in P Caplan (ed.), *The cultural construction of sexuality*, Routledge, London, pp. 52–81.

Lawson, A 2008, *Disability and equality law in Britain: the role of reasonable adjustment*, Hart Publishing, Oxford.

Levinson, J 2010, *Making life work: freedom and disability in a community group home*, University of Minnesota Press, Minneapolis.

Lindau, S T and Gavrilova, N 2010, 'Sex, health, and years of sexually active life gained due to good health: evidence from two US population based cross sectional surveys of ageing', *British Medical Journal*, vol. 340, online, doi:10.1136/bmj.c810.

Lindegaard, H and Brodersen, S 2010, 'Homespace or workspace? The use of multiple assistive technologies in private dwellings', in M Schillmeier and M Domenech (eds), *New technologies and emerging spaces of care*, Ashgate, Farnham, pp. 95–106.

McCarthy, M 1999, *Sexuality and women with learning disabilities*, Jessica Kingsley Publishers, London.

McKeon, M 2005, *The secret history of domesticity: public, private, and the division of knowledge*, Johns Hopkins University Press, Baltimore.

Mansell, J 2006, 'Deinstitutionalisation and community living: progress, problems and priorities', *Journal of Intellectual & Developmental Disability*, vol. 31, no. 2, pp. 65–76.

Morris, J 1993, *Independent lives? Community care and disabled people*, Macmillan, Basingstoke.

O'Brien, J 1994, 'Down stairs that are never your own: supporting people with developmental disabilities in their own homes', *Mental Retardation*, vol. 32, pp. 1–6.

O'Brien, P, Thesing, A, Tuck, B and Capie, A 2001, 'Perceptions of change, advantage and quality of life for people with intellectual disability who left a long stay institution to live in the community', *Journal of Intellectual & Developmental Disability*, vol. 26, no. 1, pp. 67–82.

O'Callaghan, A C and Murphy, G H 2004, 'Capacity of adults with intellectual disabilities to consent to sexual relationships', *Psychological Medicine*, vol. 34, pp. 1347–1357.

O'Callaghan, A C and Murphy, G H 2007, 'Sexual relationships in adults with intellectual disabilities: understanding the law', *Journal of Intellectual Disability Research*, vol. 51, no. 3, pp. 197–206.

OED online 2012, *Oxford English dictionary*, accessed 22 December 2012, http://oed.com.

Ozaki, Y 1900, 'Misunderstood Japan', *The North American Review*, October 1900, pp. 566–576.

Philo, C and Parr, H 2000, 'Institutional geographies: introductory remarks', *Geoforum*, vol. 31, pp. 513–521.

Reiss, S, Levitan, G W and Szyszko, J 1982, 'Emotional disturbance and mental retardation: diagnostic overshadowing', *American Journal of Mental Deficiency*, vol. 86, pp. 567–574.

Rosenblatt, P C 2006, *Two in a bed: the social system of couple bed sharing*, State University of New York Press, Albany.

Roulstone, A and Mason-Bish, H (2012) *Disability, hate crime and violence*, Routledge, London.

Shakespeare, T, Gillespie-Sells, K and Davies, D 1996, *The sexual politics of disability: untold desires*, Cassell, London.

Silver, A 1997, 'Two different sorts of commerce – friendship and strangership', in J Weintraum and K Kumar (eds), *Public and private in thought and practice: perspectives on a grand dichotomy*, Chicago University Press, Chicago, pp. 43–74.

Ulanowicz, A (n.d.), *Phillipe Aries*, accessed 3 February 2014, www.representingchildhood.pitt.edu/pdf/aries.pdf.

United Nations 2006, *United Nations Convention on the Rights of Persons with Disabilities*, United Nations General Assembly, New York.

Valentine, G 2001, *Social geographies: space and society*, Prentice Hall, Harlow.

Vislie, L 2003, 'From integration to inclusion: focusing global trends and changes in the western European societies', *European Journal of Special Needs Education*, vol. 18, no. 1, pp. 17–35.

Walmsley, J 2005, 'Institutionalization: a historical perspective', in K Johnson and R Traustadóttir (eds), *Deinstitutionalization and people with intellectual disabilities: in and out of institutions*, Jessica Kingsley Publishers, London, pp. 50–65.

Weeks, J 2012, *Sex, politics and society: the regulation of sexuality since 1800*, Longman, Harlow.

10 Eroding the collective 'places' of support

Emerging geographies of personalisation for people with intellectual disabilities

Andrew Power

Introduction

Disability policy has evolved since 2004 to a greater focus on individually-tailored supports and interventions to enable people with intellectual disabilities (referred to as learning disabilities in the UK) achieve active participation and engagement in the community. In response to the shifting policy emphasis, support environments are increasingly becoming more decentralised to enable people to live more independently, which is having implications on the way services have been designed. At the same time, there has been an accelerating erosion of state and provider-led supports and entitlements and an increasing push towards local actors and institutions in the delivery of support. New roles and a myriad of new individualised support arrangements have emerged in response to the shifting emphasis in support delivery (Dowling *et al.*, 2006). As a result, the 'local' is an increasingly important axis whereby support services are becoming configured. A geographical focus can help to unpack *where* persons with intellectual disabilities (or learning disabilities) are being supported, with a focus on their everyday environment and the extent to which they are connected. Such a focus can help uncover new spatial arrangements of support. This chapter examines these new trends, focusing on the changing landscape of support. It provides a critical socio-geographical appraisal of the emerging processes and effects of the recent disability policy context, providing insights into the complex everyday negotiations and challenges of facilitating individually-tailored support arrangements.

This more recent development has been largely driven by the philosophy of personalisation (referred to as self-determination in the United States) which seeks to enable an individual to move away from passive dependence on paternalistic, inflexible group services and an embrace of self-directed supports to promote and facilitate agency and self-determination (Algozzine *et al.*, 2001). The process of promoting personalisation means putting the individual at the centre of the process of identifying their needs and allowing them to make choices about how, when and by whom they are supported to live their lives.

The recent United Nations (UN) Convention on the Rights of Persons with Disabilities (CRPD) powerfully reinforces this new set of values. In particular,

Article 19 of the UN CRPD demands that services should be closely tied to the achievement of choice and independence as well as community involvement. It affirms that:

> States Parties to the Convention recognize the equal right of all persons with disabilities to live in the community, with choices equal to others, and shall take effective and appropriate measures to facilitate full enjoyment by persons with disabilities of this right and their full inclusion and participation in the community.
>
> (Art. 19, 2007)

Accordingly, the emphasis is not on services per se, but supports to enable active and meaningful lives in the community. Since the CRPD, the European Commission has mirrored these guiding principles, with the publication of its *European disability strategy 2010–2020: a renewed commitment to a barrier-free Europe* (2010). Its main focus has been the removal of obstacles to inclusion in order to make it easier for people with disabilities to go about their daily lives like everyone else – and enjoy their rights as citizens.

This changing policy landscape has an important influence on policy-makers interested in redesigning service delivery models, service providers interested in re-imagining their services in the decades to come and persons with intellectual disabilities anxious to ensure that future services are adequate to ensure their right to live independent lives and be included in the community. At the heart of this change is a move away from conventional models of support based on group services with limited choice towards giving people more choice and control over the support they require to live independently and participate in their community (O'Brien and Sullivan, 2005). The favouring of this approach by policy-makers is arguably linked to its close resonance with the wider neoliberal agenda of individualism, thus suggesting, on the surface at least, a mirroring of governmental and Disabled People's Movement developments towards personal autonomy and choice (Roulstone and Morgan, 2009).

At the same time, an emerging context of austerity and social care budget cuts is being seen in many countries, derived from a combination of demographic change and major pressures on public expenditure, which is having a substantial impact on the implementation of this reform agenda (Lymbery, 2012). As a result, the strongest critics of personalisation have homed in on its connections with neoliberal political ideologies and see personalisation as a cost-cutting agenda in itself (see, for example, Ferguson, 2007; Houston, 2010). While this criticism has become more pervasive, nonetheless many still see personalisation as a way of restoring people's rights as citizens (Oliver and Sapey, 2006) and for enhancing the levels of independence and autonomy of persons with disabilities (Leece and Peace, 2010).

At the heart of this debate regarding the implementation of personalisation is a reconfigured 'geography of care' in terms of the changing patterns and environments of support and the spatial outcomes which are emerging. The reconfiguration of support has had significant geographical implications on the lives of persons with intellectual disabilities and on the myriad of embedded support staff, advocates, volunteers and families which must operate within this environment (see Philo and Metzel, 2005). Rather than thinking of this geography as a fixed grid across which people are located, the chapter also considers the active role geography plays in shaping the networks and interactions involved within the support environment. According to Cutchin (2005), within geography, it is understood that places have an active role in shaping human behaviour, for example the sites of support can play a role in shaping the behaviour and routines of staff, invoke fears of parents facing the unknown in the community, confronting issues of privacy, feelings of belonging, and connection and companionship within local neighbourhoods.

To understand how personalisation and its associated landscape of support has materialised, the chapter charts the changes in how support policy has shifted since 2004 and traces the changing geography of support from this time. The chapter draws on secondary analyses of outcome evaluation research as well as my own recent fieldwork with service managers and government officials within relevant disability statutory bodies (Power, 2013), to identify and critically examine how these shifts have manifested themselves, and how different stakeholders have been repositioned in the process. This fieldwork involved site visits to British Columbia (BC) in Canada, the UK, the United States and Ireland between mid-2009 and mid-2010. The chapter draws on approaches from these different jurisdictions including emerging initiatives which have sought to meet the new policy focus by helping to broaden people's 'natural' connections within the community and live in more inclusive environments. In particular, it focuses on two evolving support models and their associated roles for different stakeholders: community connectors and home share/host families, which are seeking to fill the gaps amidst an increasing array of decentralised support arrangements. Community connectors focus on cultivating informal support arrangements in the 'ordinary' rather than 'special' places in the community, such as local recreation centres, schools, clubs, libraries and coffee shops, for example, and to facilitate associational connections and a sense of belonging within these sites (O'Brien and Sullivan, 2005). Meanwhile, home share/host families offer to 'host' a person with intellectual disabilities within their own homes as well as share family and community life together. The chapter concludes with a discussion of the different socio-spatial outcomes, challenges and risks in translating this new paradigm into a viable new landscape of support.

New geographies of social support

The following sections of the chapter examine some of the main shifts that have taken place within the social support market (known within the UK as the 'adult social care' market) in recent years, from the first wave of deinstitutionalisation to the renewed policy focus on personalisation, emphasising the geographical shifts that have taken place. To some extent, pioneering support providers allied with disability advocates have driven this change and have led the way in developing new and innovative ways to support people with intellectual disabilities. In most other cases, however, the 'conventional' support market characterised by group homes and day care settings is trying to adapt to the changing policy focus by reconfiguring their service models and support roles. As the next section shall examine, a key part of this agenda has been to re-sculpt the social ecology of persons with disabilities in an effort to create stronger networks within the community.

Re-sculpting the social ecology of persons with disabilities

Much has been written on the changing landscape of support as a result of deinstitutionalisation (Dear and Taylor, 1982). Its history as a site of care and treatment has had profound effects on persons with disabilities as well as leaving behind a legacy of expectations and attitudes regarding their ongoing dependency in service settings, as traced by many geographers (Park et al., 1998; Park and Radford, 1999; Philo, 2004). Indeed, Moon et al. argue that deinstitutionalisation was 'profoundly geographic' in the way in which it sought an end to 'the removal of the "client" from the stresses of everyday life through confinement' (2006: 131). Nonetheless, Roulstone and Morgan (2009) warn of the false binary of automatically associating collective day centre provision as a bad service model, and community support being a relative panacea. Importantly, the first wave of community care in North America saw an emerging 'landscape of despair' characterised by homelessness and ghettoisation of discharged populations into the community (Dear and Wolch, 1987).

Deinstitutionalisation paved the way for a new landscape of support centred on group homes and boarding houses, day care centres, special schools, rehabilitation, occupational therapy, special bus services and sheltered workshops. Laws and Radford (1998) traced the geographies of social care for persons with intellectual disabilities in Toronto. They found that many lived in group homes or alone in apartments, struggled with a shortage of money, and had limited social activities and social networks. Less than 30 per cent of those who had work socialised with their workmates. Overall, Laws and Radford maintained that, despite deinstitutionalisation, people with intellectual disabilities are 'particularly vulnerable to being invisible in the community' (1998: 88). Similarly in the UK, it was found by Forrester-Jones et al. (2006) that the breadth of social relationships remained low for adults with learning difficulties 12 years after they had left institutional settings. Drawing on a sample of 213 such adults, it was found that the size of the average social network for these individuals was 22 people (range 3–51), with 25 per cent being other service users, 43 per cent staff, 14 per cent family members, and 11 per cent miscellaneous others. The authors concluded that, despite being resettled from long-stay hospitals, these social networks were smaller and qualitatively different than normative social networks. More generally, group homes have been found in many cases to have similar service arrangements and care practices to larger institutions (European

Commission Ad Hoc Expert Group on the Transition from Institutional to Community-based Care, 2000).

Multiple problems have been associated with group home arrangements regardless of their size. These outcomes include: inflexible schedules, high levels of staffing, incompatibility/disputes among residents, inability to adapt to residents' changing needs/preferences, and low levels of personal choice and autonomy regarding group activities and decisions (Stancliffe and Lakin, 2005). In terms of their social ecology, relationships in these settings were less likely to be described as 'close' compared with relationships in small group homes and supported accommodation (Forrester-Jones, 1998). Research also indicates that some individuals residing in group homes do not require such high levels of support and may demonstrate better outcomes, at lower cost, by living semi-independently (Stainton *et al.*, 2006).

While this 'formal' landscape of support still exists to a large extent, generally a large proportion of adults with intellectual disabilities live at home and are being supported by their parents (see McCallion and Nickle, 2008) whilst making use of some group services and interventions, such as local day care centres, and caregiver respite centres (Beresford, 1994; Power, 2010). Many experience being tied to the home, and tend to utilise sites of 'nested dependencies' (Kittay, 1999), situational contexts where sources of support are embedded, such as neighbour's homes, or local care groups (Power, 2008). Moreover, parents often acknowledge feelings of overprotection, despite their wishes to promote more independence for their adult children with intellectual disabilities (Power, 2008).

In an effort to promote more meaningful lives in the community, person-centred planning (PCP) approaches came to dominate intellectual disability services in the mid-1990s/early 2000s, leading to a new emphasis on assisting the individual to plan their life and supports. It arose in response to ongoing dissatisfaction with the service-led approach, where people were forced to fit within particular group service models, and thereby further disempowering and excluding them (O'Brien and Lyle-O'Brien, 2006). PCP was designed specifically to place the individual at the centre of decision-making, treating family members as partners, and offer more choice and flexibility in the types of required supports offered (O'Brien and Lyle-O'Brien, 2006).

PCP has been adopted in a number of jurisdictions, including many states in the United States (Mount, 1992), in provinces across Canada (through circles of support) (Gold, 1994) and in England with the *Valuing people* White Paper (Department of Health [DoH], 2001). Evaluations in the United States (see Holburn and Vietze, 2002) revealed that the quality of life indicators of autonomy, choice-making, daily activities, relationships and satisfaction improved more for the PCP group than the contrast group. Similarly, an evaluation of PCP in the UK by Robertson *et al.* demonstrated that with PCP, people were associated with having a 52 per cent increase in size of social networks, 2.4 times greater chance of having active contact with family, 40 per cent increase in level of contact with friends and 30 per cent increase in number of community-based activities. However, it is worth bearing in mind that the results indicated a strong influence of factors relating to the characteristics of participants, contextual factors, and the type of PCP process used.

In more recent times, this process of person-centred support has evolved into person-*led* support, and has become known as the 'personalisation' or 'choice' agenda (DH, 2009). This approach focuses on self-led support, individual funding, such as direct payments or personal budgets, and an emphasis on moving away from 'conventional' services such as day care to living independently and working in the open labour market. The evolution of this policy might be viewed as the culmination of the normalisation and deinstitutionalisation movements that started in the early 1970s and a cross-fertilisation of ideas from the independent living movement, driven largely by persons with physical disabilities.

One of the core elements of personalisation has been individual funding. Evaluations of individual funding in the United States (Head and Conroy, 2005) found significant improvements in choice and control, quality of life, satisfaction and community participation, following implementation of Consumer Directed Services in Michigan. However, as yet, individual funding has not been as well-accepted or well-adopted as a model of support for persons with learning disabilities, as many find the processes involved, such as financial management and recruitment of workers, stressful (IBSEN, 2008). Moreover, a perhaps unintentional outcome of this shift has meant a gradual erosion of those sites of care associated with community care (i.e. day care centres, drop-in centres) given the decline of funding towards group care settings. Services are reframing their emphasis towards accessing 'mainstream' community amenities and facilities, rather than relying on the availability of special day services (Simpson, 2007). The use of day care centres in the UK, for example, fell within individual funding pilot sites: the average amount of time spent in day care fell from around 4.5 days per week to 3.5 days per week per person (Bartlett, 2009). More generally, day centres providing activities and support for disabled people are closing, as budgets are reduced, and providing support within collective spaces, local amenities and facilities within mainstream community settings is increasingly seen as the appropriate scale of caring (*Guardian*, 2010).This erosion of day services, according to Roulstone and Morgan (2009), raises important questions over whether the reduced opportunities to meet in group settings is undermining the social networks and collective identity of people with learning disabilities. They found that with self-directed support many users end up spending a great deal of former centre-based time at home and not having the quantity of financial support required to allow them to engage freely with other disabled people and the wider public.

This trend will likely continue, resulting in an increasingly 'place-less' service landscape, which has significant implications for persons with intellectual disabilities traditionally using site-based services, and for practitioners and support staff who are being called upon to work in an increasingly decentralised support environment. For individuals, there are therefore potentially new opportunities with personalisation, but also the potential for social and spatial isolation, with the gradual erosion of conventional sites of support and limited social ecology networks. The following section thus examines in more detail two models of support which have evolved within the current context of personalisation.

Responding to decentralised lives

Given the contemporary disability support landscape characterised above, a new generation of service delivery models has begun to fill the gaps in terms of supporting people outside of conventional service arrangements. This section looks at two emerging strands of service provision: community connection and home share/host families, with a renewed focus on generating a new 'geography of care', by linking people together, connecting to the community and reshaping roles for support workers, volunteers and families.

One of the first strands has been the role of community connection within disability services. This type of role was developed initially in British Columbia by organisations such as the PLAN Institute, which established a model where 'community connectors' cultivate linkages with persons in the community who have similar interests to the person with the disability. They locate these connections within social clubs, associations, local businesses, churches and other faith communities, colleges and universities; indeed, anywhere there may be a potential person who could develop a friendship or relationship with the disabled person. With this model, rather than simply re-placing people back into the community, the work of support staff is focused on having to carefully develop linkages with people in the community. Those involved in support also must pay attention to the community calendar of events to utilise key places at particular times, for example local fêtes, festivals, concerts, etc.

Community connectors have since been used by many other providers in Canada and other jurisdictions including the UK and Ireland. Importantly, the types of support roles within such providers are increasingly not confined to personal care. In the UK, within an organisation called Keyring, for example, which has the same ethos of promoting community connections, the essential requirements for support worker jobs now includes the 'ability to talk easily to people such as neighbours and families and agencies' (Keyring, 2013). In addition, staff are required to 'build up links with local people and organisations and to encourage members to make use of good will, neighbourliness, and facilities in their community'; 'to offer support in a flexible and creative way when needed'; 'to see members in the evenings and the weekends'; 'to organize one's work time in a flexible way' (Keyring, 2013).

Within this new decentralised landscape of support, more complex negotiations amongst staff, families and volunteers are often required. According to service provider managers and government officials with relevant disability portfolios, recognising the challenges in cultivating a sense of cohesion, reciprocity and belonging for adults with intellectual disabilities within the local neighbourhood can be a delicate process. Recognising family anxieties about this new geography of support and building up trust is often a challenge which support providers must grapple with, particularly for parents who have experienced first-hand previous policy commitments to group homes and day care services:

> What we found with families was managing, not only managing expectations, but managing how they were feeling about us presenting an option to them

around their family person not being in a congregated service and dealing with their feelings about having to do that in the first place. There was a lot of anxiety and guilt about what had happened (with deinstitutionalisation) and for us to then come all these years later and say – 'you know what … we're moving to this new model', that was really difficult for some families … If we were able to help parents talk to others who had gone through that, and alleviate the fear … there's a long way to changing that.

(Government official, British Columbia)

Moreover, there is an increasing recognition of the complex and active role space and place plays in considering support arrangements and in unbundling group services. The level of 'unknowns' associated with a life in the community was a shared concern amongst all relevant stakeholders:

Life is complex, and so living in the community is complex, and it's not black and white, it really does depend on the structures, and the safeguards and all the kind of things you put in place to help people to have a quality of life. And if people are willing to sort of figure that out and have more questions than answers but take the time to do that, then you are way better ahead.

(Same government official, British Columbia)

In an effort to ease these fears about achieving feelings of inclusion in the community, the model of community connection involves a certain amount of 'social interpretation', a concept which recognises that many persons with intellectual disabilities often need support to understand an increasingly complex cognitive world (O'Brien and Sullivan, 2005). The social interpreter role is designed to assist the person to understand what is happening in their environment, assist them to make the decisions they wish to take and assist them to exercise their rights (National Advisory Committee on Health and Disability, 2003: 21). This can be complex work and can involve delicate negotiations with members of the public:

It takes a while to be set up. Bridging connections between folks, helping start conversations and guiding our volunteers, there's a lot of trust building that goes on between our clients and the public. Here in the community centre, there's a lot of subtle work going on in the background to ensure the public feel comfortable coming in and using the facilities [with our clients]. And easing any fears or insecurities involved. And our clients run the café. So bit by bit there's barriers being broken down and more of our clients are feeling part of their community. But you can't expect these things to just happen by themselves. With the cutbacks, our advocates are getting less and less hours to do this work.

(Service manager, Ireland)

Recognising the challenges above in bridging connections and easing fears amongst clients and members of the public appears to be an important aspect of support work tailored towards facilitating independent living in the community. This type of work represents an important shift in emphasis from 'doing for a person' to assisting a person to make informed decisions as opposed to having their lives misunderstood and restricted. Moreover, this is an important shift given that often persons with intellectual disabilities are not as socially connected with friends and allies, given their often limited social ecology networks, making it harder for them to make decisions about their lives. This function therefore is something which should become routine in the fabric of the support environment.

A second support model evolving within this geography of support has been the Home Share/Host Family model which has developed widely in Canada and Ireland, amongst other countries. The Home Share model initially emerged in the mid-1980s on quite a limited basis as a way of enabling people without close family ties to live in more inclusive environments. It normally involved a less intensive living arrangement for persons with mild intellectual disabilities with good independent living skills where they share a tenancy or owner-occupied home with another individual or family. More recently, a variant has developed called the Host Family model, which is a supported living arrangement where a broader range of individuals with disabilities (including those classified as 'profound') live either full-time or for a fixed number of nights per week with a host family or individual. Each approved host family agrees contractually to provide a specific number of respite sessions per month. For both variants, an allowance is paid for each host person depending on level of need and the length of the session whether weekday or weekend (Brothers of Charity Galway [BOCG], 2009). There are also many variants to the types of contracts settled, as illustrated by the quote from a service provider below, including options for tax free allowance, retainers, and free rent for renters.

> We paid a grant to the support worker [host person], set approximately at care assistant rates, but built in flexibility in her hours and built in respite options. We put a package together of €30,000 to be paid to the family, which we took out of her group home budget. So we made a contract with the family over monitoring visits and it was decided that the whole family would need to get police background clearance.
>
> (Service provider, Ireland)

The Host Family model is designed to fit alongside more conventional service interventions such as supported employment or personal assistance in the home. According to a pilot of this model, called 'Contract Families' in Galway, Ireland, it was found to provide a cost-effective alternative to residential services, with resources used to better effect and the provision of a better quality of support overall (BOCG, 2009).

However, setting up these contract families is often a difficult process in terms of building up trust amongst individuals who have been in conventional care settings for some time and their older parents.

Some of the individuals that we're supporting differently, because they've come from a context of driving the change because things were so bad for them and they were so unhappy, there's a lot of trust that has been damaged over the years so it's not like we're all sitting around a circle of support and it's all happy-clappy. It's very tense. And it can be very difficult at times. And it can take many years of working together to try and rebuild the trust. And the only way we can do it is not to keep reminding families how nice we are. They want to see real evidence that we're doing what we said on the team, that we're giving them the control, that we're giving them the money or doing things differently. Whatever it might be.

(Service provider, Ireland)

Matching individuals to hosts is becoming an important function for support providers. Many intellectual disability services now have dedicated host family coordinators, to organise recruitment events to recruit, screen and hire host persons; manage administration, facilitation and coordination of activities; work with the individual to design a personalised living preference plan; and liaise with the multidisciplinary team to ensure the individual's support needs are met. According to the Galway pilot:

Recruiting suitable families for this type of care work will continue to be very time consuming and labour intensive, particularly at Social Worker level, though the back-up administrative support will also prove crucial … It has and will create the need to find, assess, train, and approve replacement families, so as to maintain and develop current levels of service.

(BOCG, 2009: 4)

For this reason, a separate host family coordinator role is often established with clear terms of reference, particularly with respect to management and delegated authority functions.

These two models have sought to provide important sources of support at the margins within a new and emerging era of personalisation. The multifaceted socio-spatial dimensions of these responses to this social policy are explored for persons with disabilities, families, staff and managers in the following discussion.

Discussion

Personalisation now lies at the heart of social policy in the jurisdictions examined in this chapter. Given the powerful reinforcement of its guiding principles in the UN Convention and other regional policies, it is likely to continue to lead to reform of social support (Tyson *et al.*, 2010). Geographically, personalisation has led increasingly to a move away from financial and political investment in collective level care provision (Kastner and Walsh, 2008), and to an increasing reliance on the interdependent networks of 'natural' support from (host) families, carers and organisations within which people with intellectual disabilities live their everyday lives. Adult social care has therefore arguably evolved from a context of deinstitutionalisation to one of de-service-isation, characterised by attempts to enable people with intellectual disabilities to have more meaningful lives in the community, albeit within an increasingly fragile and decentralised support environment.

Taking on board this broader context, this section provides a discussion of the different geographic and socio-relational outcomes, risks and challenges in translating this new paradigm of support into workable models of service delivery. It considers the implications of these broader shifts on the ground, since the initial roots of reform from deinstitutionalisation, centred on the practices and experiences of those involved in developing these new support models. At this scale, it is possible to see the active role of geography in shaping the experiences, hopes, fears and negotiations of support workers, families, support managers, and ultimately the individuals themselves, in the process of shaping these new support arrangements.

In terms of socio-spatial outcomes and challenges for the support workforce, support workers may be increasingly required to have an active knowledge of the local community, identifying welcoming spaces and unwelcoming sites, and be involved in correspondence and outreach work to encourage independent living in the community. In effect, support staff, host family coordinators and host families themselves are being asked to map on their support to the local geography and embed care within neighbourhood networks, by drawing on and building up links with local people and organisations and by encouraging clients to make use of goodwill, neighbourliness and facilities in their community. The move away from care provision being confined to personal care roles and a related shift in the balance of power will therefore undoubtedly lead to a reshaping of boundaries.

There are also socio-spatial challenges for families in accepting and facing the unknown in the community, particularly for those who have previously been advised that a group home or day care centre was the best place for their adult son or daughter. These fears of the unknown in the local neighbourhood resonate with geographic work on the complex coding of spaces of inclusion/exclusion, particularly for marginalised groups. As Hall (2005) notes, 'persons with intellectual disabilities often face a "double-bind" of marginalisation, experiencing exclusion *from* and discrimination *within* the very social spaces that are the key markers of social inclusion policy' (p. 110). More generally, marginalised people can be made to feel 'out-of-place' in locations where their presence is seen to disrupt the norms, values and behaviours of that place (Cresswell, 1996). Consequently, promoting the idea of a meaningful life in the community to parents of adults with intellectual disabilities is a process which must be considered carefully.

In terms of challenges for support managers, it is clear that despite positive outcomes being documented in pilots of personalisation (Stainton *et al.*, 2009), in order for this transformation to successfully enable more persons to have meaningful lives in the community, the process will require the exercise of strong and collective leadership by managers. In particular, these leadership skills will be required to bring about the kinds of service level infrastructure that might be needed to sustain such an approach, given the management and administrative issues (Kendrick and Sullivan, 2009). There will be an increased volume of persons involved in care coordination work, as well as wider coordination with family, volunteers, home share hosts, and so on. According to the Social Care Institute for Excellence (2009) in the UK, providers have stated that the most significant changes will include trying to change attitudes and ways of working, improving status for care staff, offering new ways to deliver care, and providing localised teams to ensure consistency.

Finally, despite the best intentions of these new support models, taking on board the above considerations, there remains a serious potential risk for individuals with intellectual disabilities of becoming more exposed to isolation, abuse or being wholly dependent on already constrained natural supports if the evolving support landscape is not managed carefully. With both models, there is often an implicit assumption that building individual and family capacity to support a person can lead to a reduction in the need for services. Promoting the resilience of families and local allies through community connection and personalisation should not simply translate to a lesser role for government in supporting adult social care, as illuminated by the quote below from a former advocate of the community living movement and current service provider manager in British Columbia:

> So the dilemma is, an exclusive focus on personalisation without understanding the economic, political and social context we're in, in the twenty-first century whether we're in BC or in other countries, I think risks jeopardising a lot of what we have. I don't personally believe that we've made enough advances in human rights for people with disabilities that we can guarantee that Triage won't happen again, a new wave of eugenics won't happen, I think there's already what I call a new worthiness – I think there is already – and it's been around for quite some time, a policy consideration that you won't hear front and centre but is in the background, about who is more worthy than others who are receiving government support. And so all of those make me really concerned.
>
> (Service manager, British Columbia)

Taking these concerns on board, the role of the state and those involved in commissioning adult social care remains critical in terms of making sure there are standards and safeguards in place, rather than community living and personalisation being seen solely as a cost-saving exercise. Given the broader context discussed above, it will require careful and responsible governance to ensure people do not become entirely de-coupled from support services without allied support networks being put in place.

Conclusion

The way in which personalisation has challenged a long history of paternalism that has characterised social care leaves little doubt that persons with disabilities have valued the extent to which the levels of independence and autonomy are enhanced by personalisation. In particular, personalisation has the potential to radically change the way in which persons with intellectual disabilities receive services as well as improve the values-based context within which they live their everyday lives. Mirroring the development of personalisation, however, is an erosion of conventional services. How this process evolves will remain a challenge for all stakeholders involved in providing support, with many risks and potentially harmful impacts for individuals and their families. How this process is managed to ensure these risks are minimised will be crucial. Future research therefore needs to continue contributing to understanding the scope and limitations of personalisation policies in terms of how they play out across space and place in order to help address these complex challenges, and to encourage the transfer of knowledge between all the stakeholders concerned. With an appreciation of the socio-spatial challenges of implementing personalisation within the current context of austerity, it is no longer acceptable to uncritically champion this approach, without laying open the processes of implementation to closer scrutiny.

References

Algozzine, B, Browder, D, Karvonen, M, Test, D W and Wood, W M 2001, 'Effects of interventions to promote self-determination for individuals with disabilities', *Review of Educational Research*, vol. 71, no. 2, pp. 219–277.

Bartlett, J 2009, *At your service: navigating the future market in health and social care*, Demos, London.

Beresford, B 1994, *Positively parents: caring for a severely disabled child*, University of York, Social Policy Research Unit, York.

Brothers of Charity Galway (BOCG) 2009, *Room for one more: contract families pilot scheme 07-09 evaluation report*, Brothers of Charity Galway, Galway.

Cresswell, T 1996, *In place/out of place*, University of Minnesota Press, Minnesota.

Cutchin, M P, 2005, 'Spaces for inquiry into the role of place for older people's care', *International Journal of Older People Nursing in association with Journal of Clinical Nursing*, vol. 14, no. 8b, pp. 121–129.

Dear, M and Taylor, S M 1982, *Not on our street: community attitudes to mental health care*, Pion, London.

Dear, M and Wolch, J 1987, *Landscapes of despair: from deinstitutionalization to homelessness*, Polity Press, Cambridge.

Department of Health (DoH) 2001, *Valuing people*, HM Government, London.

Department of Health (DoH) 2009, Transforming adult social care: local authority circular, HM Government, London.

Dowling, S, Manthorpe, J and Cowley, S 2006, *Person-centred planning in social care – an exploration of the relevance of person-centred planning in social care: a scoping review*, Joseph Rowntree Foundation, York.

European Commission 2010, *European disability strategy 2010–2020: a renewed commitment to a barrier-free Europe*, 15 November 2010, European Commission, Brussels.

European Commission Ad Hoc Expert Group on the Transition from Institutional to Community-based Care 2000, *Report of the ad hoc expert group on the transition from institutional to community-based care*, European Commission, Brussels.

Ferguson, I 2007, 'Increasing user choice or privatizing risk? The antinomies of personalisation', *British Journal of Social Work*, vol. 37, no. 3, pp. 387–403.

Forrester-Jones, R 1998, 'Social networks and social support: development of instrument', Departmental Working Paper, Tizard Centre, University of Kent at Canterbury, *Disability and Society*, vol. 13, pp. 389–413.

Forrester-Jones, R, Carpenter, J, Coolen-Schrijner, P, Cambridge, P, Tate, A, Beecham, J, Hallam, A, Knapp, M and Wooff, D 2006, 'The social networks of people with intellectual disability living in the community 12 years after resettlement from long-stay hospitals', *Journal of Applied Research in Intellectual Disabilities*, vol. 19, pp. 285–295.

Gold, D 1994, '"We don't call it a 'circle'": the ethos of a support group', *Disability and Society*, vol. 9, no. 4, pp. 435–452.

Guardian 2010, 'Birmingham city council to cut up to 2000 jobs and close care homes', 10 February.

Hall, E 2005, 'Entangled geographies of inclusion/exclusion for adults with learning disabilities', *Health & Place*, vol. 11, no. 2, pp. 107–115.

Head, M J and Conroy, J W 2005, 'Outcomes of self-determination in Michigan: quality and costs', in R J Stancliffe and K C Lakin (eds), *Costs and outcomes of community services for people with intellectual disabilities*, Paul H. Brookes Publishing, Baltimore, pp. 219–240.

Holburn, S and Vietze, P (eds) 2002, *Person-centered planning: research, practice and future directions*, Paul H. Brookes, Baltimore.

Houston, S 2010, 'Beyond homo economicus: recognition and self-realization and social work', *British Journal of Social Work*, vol. 40, no. 3, pp. 841–857.

IBSEN 2008, *Evaluation of the individual budgets pilot programme*, University of York, Social Policy Research Unit, York.

Kastner, T and Walsh, K 2008, 'Divided we stand, united we fall: personal budgets versus universal coverage', *Intellectual and Developmental Disabilities*, vol. 46, no. 3, pp. 239–242.

Kendrick, M and Sullivan, L 2009, 'Appraising the leadership challenges of social inclusion', *The International Journal of Leadership in Public Services*, vol. 5, pp. 67–75.

Keyring 2013, *Paid support opportunities*, Keyring, London, accessed 14 May 2013, www.keyring.org/site/KEYR/Templates/Generic3col.aspx?pageid=197&cc=GB.

Kittay, E 1999, *Love's labour: essays on women, equality and dependency*, Routledge, New York.

Laws, G and Radford, J 1998, 'Place, identity and disability: narratives of intellectually disabled people', in R Kearns and W Gesler (eds), *Putting health into place: landscape, identity and well-being*, Syracuse University Press, Syracuse, pp. 77–101.

Leece, J and Peace, S 2010, 'Developing new understandings of independence and autonomy in the personalised relationship', *British Journal of Social Work*, vol. 40, no. 6, pp. 1847–1865.

Lymbery, M 2012, 'Social work and personalisation', *British Journal of Social Work*, vol. 42, no. 4, pp. 783–792.

McCallion, P and Nickle, T 2008, 'Individuals with developmental disabilities and their caregivers', *Journal of Gerontological Social Work*, 50 (SUPP/1), pp. 245–266.

Moon, G, Kearns, R and Joseph, A 2006, 'Selling the private asylum: therapeutic landscapes and the (re)valorization of confinement in the era of community care', *Transactions of the Institute of British Geographers*, vol. 31, pp. 131–149.

Mount, B 1992, *Person centred planning: a sourcebook of values, ideas and methods to encourage person-centered development*, Graphic Futures, New York.

National Advisory Committee on Health and Disability 2003, *To have an 'ordinary life'*, a report to the Minister of Health and the Minister for Disability Issues, NACHD, New Zealand.

O'Brien, J and Lyle-O'Brien, C 2006, *Implementing person centred planning: voices of experience*, Inclusion Press, Toronto.

O'Brien, P and Sullivan, M 2005, *Allies in emancipation: moving from providing service to being of support*, Thomson Dunmore, South Melbourne.

Oliver, M and Sapey, B 2006, *Social work with disabled people*, 3rd edn, Palgrave, Basingstoke.

Park, D and Radford, J 1999, 'Rhetoric and place in the "mental deficiency" asylum', in R Butler and H Parr (eds), *Mind and body spaces: geographies of illness, impairment and disability*, Routledge, London, pp. 69–96.

Park, D, Radford, J and Vickers, M 1998, 'Disability studies in human geography', *Progress in Human Geography*, vol. 22, no. 2, pp. 208–233.

Philo, C 2004, *The space reserved for insanity: a geographical history of institutional provision for the insane from medieval times to the 1860s in England and Wales*, Edwin Mellen Press, Lewiston, Queenston and Lampeter.

Philo, C and Metzel, D 2005, 'Editorial: introduction to theme section on geographies of intellectual disability: "outside the participatory mainstream"', *Health & Place (theme section on Geographies of Intellectual Disability)*, vol. 11, pp. 77–85.

Power, A 2008, 'Caring for independent lives: geographies of caring for young adults with intellectual disabilities', *Social Science & Medicine*, vol. 67, no. 5, pp. 834–843.

Power, A 2010, *Landscapes of care: comparative perspectives on family caregiving*, Ashgate, Aldershot.

Power, A 2013, *Active citizenship and disability: implementing the personalisation of support*, Cambridge University Press, New York.

Robertson, J M, Emerson, E, Hatton, C, Elliott, J, McIntosh, B, Swift, P, Krinjen-Kemp, E, Towers, C, Romeo, R, Knapp, M, Sanderson, H, Routledge, M, Oakes, P and Joyce, T 2005, *The Impact of Person Centred Planning*, Lancaster University, Division of Health Research.

Roulstone, A and Morgan, H 2009, 'Neo-liberal individualism or self-directed support: are we all speaking the same language on modernising adult social care?', *Social Policy and Society*, vol. 8, no. 3, pp. 333–345.

Simpson, M 2007, 'Community-based day services for adults with intellectual disabilities in the UK: a review and discussion', *Journal of Policy and Practice in Intellectual Disability*, vol. 4, no. 4, pp. 235–240.

Social Care Institute for Excellence (SCIE) 2009, *Personalisation briefing: implications for home care providers (At a Glance 7)*, June 2009, accessed 14 May 2013, www.scie.org.uk/publications/ataglance/ataglance07.pdf.

Stainton, T, Boyce, S and Phillips, C 2009, 'Independence pays: a cost and resource analysis of direct payments in two local authorities', *Disability and Society*, vol. 24, no. 2, pp. 161–172.

Stainton, T, Hole, R, Charles, G, Yodanis, C, Powell, S and Crawford, C 2006, *Residential options for adults with developmental disabilities: quality and cost outcomes*, October 2006, The Ministry of Children and Family Development, Province of British Columbia.

Stancliffe, R J and Lakin, K C (eds) 2005, *Costs and outcomes of community services for people with intellectual disabilities*, Paul H. Brookes, Baltimore.

Tyson, A, Brewis, R, Crosby, N, Hatton, C, Stansfield, J, Tomlinson, C, Waters, J and Wood, A 2010, *A report on In Control's third phase 2008–2009*, In Control, London.

Index

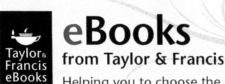

eBooks
from Taylor & Francis

Helping you to choose the right eBooks for your Library

Add to your library's digital collection today with Taylor & Francis eBooks. We have over 45,000 eBooks in the Humanities, Social Sciences, Behavioural Sciences, Built Environment and Law, from leading imprints, including Routledge, Focal Press and Psychology Press.

Choose from a range of subject packages or create your own!

Benefits for you
- Free MARC records
- COUNTER-compliant usage statistics
- Flexible purchase and pricing options
- 70% approx of our eBooks are now DRM-free.

Benefits for your user
- Off-site, anytime access via Athens or referring URL
- Print or copy pages or chapters
- Full content search
- Bookmark, highlight and annotate text
- Access to thousands of pages of quality research at the click of a button.

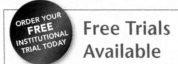

Free Trials Available

ORDER YOUR FREE INSTITUTIONAL TRIAL TODAY

We offer free trials to qualifying academic, corporate and government customers.

eCollections
Choose from 20 different subject eCollections, including:

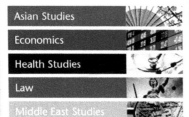

Asian Studies
Economics
Health Studies
Law
Middle East Studies

eFocus
We have 16 cutting-edge interdisciplinary collections, including:

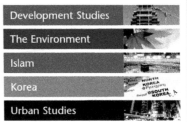

Development Studies
The Environment
Islam
Korea
Urban Studies

For more information, pricing enquiries or to order a free trial, please contact your local sales team:

UK/Rest of World: **online.sales@tandf.co.uk**
USA/Canada/Latin America: **e-reference@taylorandfrancis.com**
East/Southeast Asia: **martin.jack@tandf.com.sg**
India: **journalsales@tandfindia.com**

www.tandfebooks.com